By Beth Shaw

The YogaFit Athlete

YogaLean

Beth Shaw's YogaFit

the
yogafit® athlete

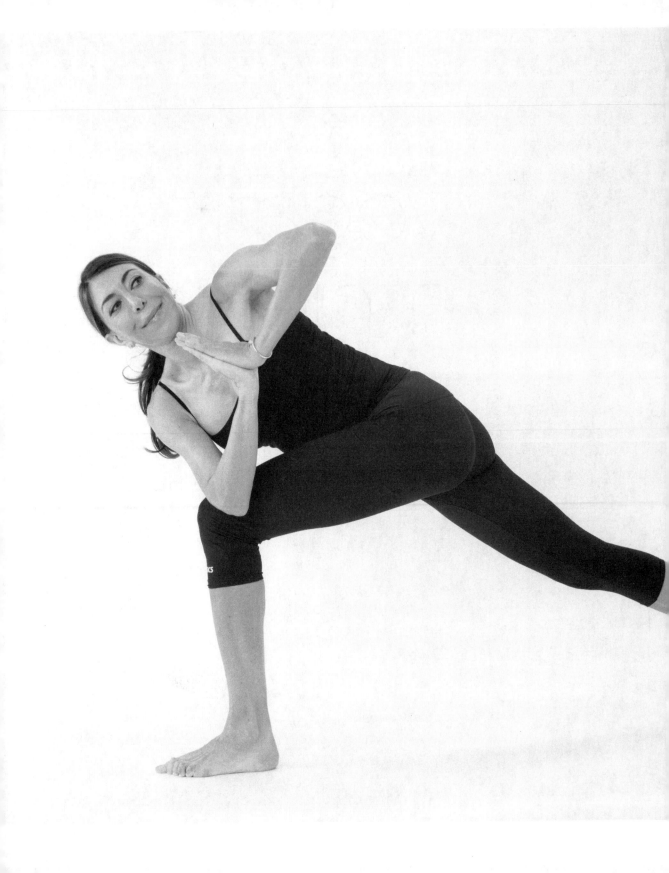

the
yogafit®
athlete

UP YOUR GAME with SPORT-SPECIFIC POSES to BUILD STRENGTH, FLEXIBILITY, and BALANCE

Beth Shaw

BALLANTINE BOOKS

NEW YORK

This book proposes a program of diet and exercise recommendations for the reader to follow. However, you should consult a qualified medical professional (and, if you are pregnant, your ob/gyn) before starting this or any other fitness program. Please seek your doctor's advice before making any decisions that affect your health or extreme changes in your diet, particularly if you suffer from any medical condition or have any symptom that may require treatment. As with any diet or exercise program, if at any time you experience any discomfort, stop immediately and consult your physician.

A Ballantine Books Trade Paperback Original

Copyright © 2016 by Beth Shaw

All rights reserved.

Published in the United States by Ballantine Books,
an imprint of Random House,
a division of Penguin Random House LLC, New York.

BALLANTINE and the HOUSE colophon are
registered trademarks of Penguin Random House LLC.

LIBRARY OF CONGRESS CATALOGING-IN-PUBLICATION DATA
Names: Shaw, Beth author.
Title: The yogafit athlete : up your game with sport-specific poses to
Build strength, flexibility, and balance / Beth Shaw.
Description: New York : Ballantine Books, 2016. | Includes index.
Identifiers: LCCN 2015049999 (print) | LCCN 2016008591 (ebook) |
ISBN 9780804178570 (paperback) | ISBN 9780804178587 (ebook)
Subjects: LCSH: Hatha yoga. | Physical fitness | BISAC: HEALTH &
FITNESS / Yoga. | HEALTH & FITNESS / Exercise. |
SPORTS & RECREATION / Reference.
Classification: LCC RA781.7 .S4463 2016 (print) | LCC RA781.7 (ebook)|
DDC 613.7/046—dc23
LC record available at http://lccn.loc.gov/2015049999

Printed in the United States of America on acid-free paper

246897531

Photographs by David Young-Wratt

Book design by Barbara M. Bachman

This is dedicated to your inner athlete.
May it flourish and shine.

CONTENTS

INTRODUCTION

Whether you're a morning jogger or a marathoner, a U.S. Open contender or just a reliable tennis partner, you're an athlete. In fact, no matter how you try to stay in shape—if you're training for the pros or a weekend warrior, if you have a sport you love—you're an athlete. Being an athlete is about more than competition. It is a commitment to a craft, focusing both mental and physical energy on honing a skill, developing a healthy and strong body, and always striving to become better.

I teach yoga, fitness, wellness, and meditation and am the founder of YogaFit, the largest yoga teacher certification program in North America, which trains people in the YogaFit and YogaLean approach. For the past twenty years, I've taught the yoga lifestyle and principles to thousands of people around the world. Yoga is a gift to the body and the mind, and my intent is to lead the way toward fitness, conscious business, and karmic responsibility. And now, I hope to help you approach your sport, whatever that may be, in a new, deeper way.

I've always been an active person—besides practicing yoga, I love swimming, running, weight training, tennis, hiking, and walking. I also work with professional athletes and coaches for the NFL. And every day as a businesswoman and role model, I'm required to show up in prime mental and physical condition.

We are all athletes in this game called life, and I encourage you to define yourself as one, too, to improve your lifestyle and physical and mental strength. An athlete's well-rounded health regimen brings them resilience and vitality in all aspects of life, not just their sport. Athletes eat and train, rather than diet and exercise. Building a sound health routine will help you navigate away from the unhealthy, unhappy, and unfit version of yourself and master your physical and mental self. This doesn't mean that you have to run a marathon or be a power lifter, but you may start to get more personally competitive and truly care for the beautiful body with which you have been gifted.

Being an athlete is a lifestyle, one that I try to live every day. My life, like so many of yours, is a race, and I want to be in the best condition I can. I'm athletic in the way I commit myself to my physical and mental health. If there's a day that I'm not active, I feel despondent, depressed, and just "off." I eat for energy and make sure that my day involves exercise. Imagine if we all lived like athletes: We would make our health our number one priority; commit to being fit and ready for action; use food as fuel and not as a vice; refrain from behaviors like smoking and drinking that move us away from a healthy lifestyle; work out regularly; strive for goals, purpose, focus, and discipline; and use mind-body techniques like meditation and visualization to achieve success.

Whether it's about work, caring for your children, being a good partner and friend, or taking care of your pets, every corner of your life is enhanced by you BEING YOUR BEST YOU. In this book, you will learn breathing exercises, physical (hatha) yoga postures appropriate to help you improve in particular sports, and three categories of poses that will augment your play in *any* sport: core/balance poses, restorative poses, and poses to be done with weights. My breathing techniques as well as mental techniques—meditation and guided imagery—complement the physical. The combination gives you many options to create your own personal plan for success.

So how do you apply yourself as an athlete? Think for a moment about how you spend most of your time. Is it at work? With your family? Regardless of your arena, chances are you want to perform at an optimum level. Athletes commit themselves to daily practices, whether it's on the field with a team, in the gym with a trainer, or in rest and recuperation. They work out regularly to gain muscle and stamina, to prevent injury, and, of course, to be better than the next. Because competition at all levels requires a fine-tuned commitment, many athletes train throughout the year to maintain excellent form, technique, and peak physical condition.

And here's my point: Athletes who are not practicing yoga are competing at a disadvantage and missing an opportunity for peak performance and longevity. The fact is that exercise tightens up your body, often putting muscle groups in opposition, and it's crucial to find a balance as well as a way to release the strain and tension in your muscles. Yoga enhances alignment, balance, core stability, strength, flexibility, agility, endurance, and mobility. It stretches muscles for greater flexibility and strengthens the core and smaller muscles, which improves form and leads to an economy of movement that significantly improves performance. It develops your lung capacity, which helps sustain a steady breath during physical activities. Lastly, yoga gives you incredible body awareness.

The sport-specific yoga poses in part II will complement your sport, enhance your performance, and reduce the risk of injury. As you fine-tune your swing or shot or general form, you are at the same time building up a "strong side." Consistent body movements, as in any sport, create habitual tightness in our muscles, often favoring one side or taxing tendons and ligaments. Here, you'll learn to build a well-balanced body by incorporating yoga throughout your weekly routine. Once a week is good; three times is better; but if you're able to weave yoga into your life as a regular routine or restorative up to five times a week, that is best. In this book, I will prescribe different regimens based on pre-season preparation, off-season maintenance, and restoring after an injury. When yoga's many benefits become part of your lifestyle, your game—and your life—will change for the better.

Just as important as the physical, athletes need acute mental concentration and focus. I know that committing daily to a very specific regimen is not easy. It takes mental balance to integrate a well-rounded practice and diet, to focus, in the moment, on making the right move and tuning out distractions. Yoga, in all its many forms, will create positive change in your mind. You'll learn meditation for greater focus, improved performance, and less stress from competing, however it is that you do it. Visualization also helps you create the winning results you desire, while what I've called "transformational language" will help you communicate with yourself in a more positive way. Positive changes add up just like negative ones do, and yoga will help eliminate the noise so that whether you compete with others or against yourself, you'll learn to set goals, develop focus, and achieve your personal best. And, most excitingly, your game will improve. One of my doctors, an avid golfer, once asked me if he should start doing yoga. He described himself as an "older, inflexible man," and I told him the same thing I tell everyone: "Yoga meets you where you live." No matter your age, flexibility level, or hobby, yoga *will* assist you. It's a process like any other—it gets better the more of it you do, and if you commit yourself, you will see and, most important, *feel* results.

the underpinnings of yoga

In the last twenty years, yoga has exploded in popularity. But yoga has been around for centuries; it's only "new" to Westerners. Yoga combines a wealth of practices that build a better body and a stronger mind using physical movement, breath control, and meditative focus. When it emerged in India more than six thousand years ago, it was aimed to train the body to sit still and meditate for long periods of time—imagine that mental strength! Over time, it became a system of psychological and physical practices to create greater health, mental awareness, and balance. Different forms and techniques evolved; at YogaFit and in this book, we teach the "hatha yoga tradition of the vinyasa style."

Hatha is a Sanskrit word that translates to "force" or "physical," but it can be broken down poetically into *ha* and *tha*. *Ha* represents the masculine, solar, or energizing qualities, and *tha* represents the feminine, lunar, or relaxing qualities. Hatha invokes the balance of opposites. The technique of vinyasa, meanwhile, means "to place in a special way," and Yoga-Fit focuses on linking poses together to create strength, flexibility, endurance, and balance.

We create classes that work all parts of the body equally, and I've designed pose sequences that trigger the body specifically based on the way it is used in a sport. Since many traditional exercise programs often overwork certain muscle groups or build muscle bulk unevenly, they tend to neglect efficient breathing or the focus on improving one's mental game. We'll strengthen the parts of the body that do not receive attention from your sport in order to develop a wholesome and well-rounded regimen. With yoga, you'll learn to expand your focus and physical practice to build more than just muscular strength.

Yoga and Flow

Flow state is a term coined by psychologist Mihaly Csikszentmihalyi in his book *Flow: The Psychology of Optimal Experience.* It means that your entire mind, body, and spirit are connected in a deep focus in order to hone in on a single activity, such as throwing a pitch or doing a pull-up. When you are in a flow state, you feel strong, alert, in effortless control, unself-conscious, and at the peak of your abilities. For instance, if you are in a flow state during a free throw shot, both mind and body are committed, which allows you to escape distractions, pressures, negative burdens, and the hecklers in the stands. Yoga and meditation balance the right and left sides of your brain to help you create these moments of full concentration and peace.

Our brains are very complex, and each part plays an important role:

- The left brain is responsible for our conscious awareness and our thoughts.
- The right brain is responsible for our creativity.
- The midbrain is responsible for the energy that powers us through the tasks of the day and for the creation of memories; it also processes real or imagined emotions.
- The brainstem is responsible for physical stimulus responses, such as swinging a bat or lacing up our running shoes.

When these four parts aren't in agreement on an objective, that objective becomes more difficult to achieve. It's like a football team where each player is running a different play. Once you get all four parts of the brain into agreement, you will have made major progress. A regular yoga practice—even just the handful of exercises and breathing techniques I will teach you in this book—will greatly enhance your ability to tap into a "flow state."

> Yoga means addition—addition of energy, strength and beauty to body, mind and soul.
>
> **—Amit Ray**

Yoga also offers a reprieve from the stresses of sports-related activities. Its poses enhance strength, cardiovascular condition, balance, and flexibility, and it creates emotional stability and reduces tightness and fatigue through mindfulness, fluid movement, and deep breathing. It massages the skeletal system that supports bone mass and growth and takes the stress away from the supporting muscles and tendons. Doesn't that sound like something that would help you before and after your daily or weekly devotion to your sport?

Imagine that you're back on that free throw line in a tied playoff game with only one minute left on the clock. How do you react? How do you focus on your shot rather than the noise and pressure? It's not easy; in fact, it's incredibly distressing. It's my goal to foster a sense of peace during high-pressure moments like those to take you gracefully through your day. Yoga, in its most simple form, is breathing and feeling. Once you achieve the physical *asanas* (poses) and focus on the mat, your mind and body will naturally translate these ideas into your every day, both on the court and off.

The Fundamentals of the YogaFit Approach

CHAPTER 1

Gaining Physical and Mental Strength Through YogaFit

The impact of yoga is never purely physical. Asanas, if correctly practiced, bridge the divide between the physical and the mental spheres. Yoga stems the feelings of pain, fatigue, doubt, confusion, indifference, laziness, self-delusion, and despair that assail us from time to time. . . . Yoga illuminates your life. If you practice sincerely, with seriousness and honesty, its light will spread to all aspects of your life.

—B.K.S. Iyengar

verall body strength is a building block of success regardless of your sport or athletic activity. No amount of weight lifting with free weights will give you the strength that is achieved by holding up your own body weight in yoga. (Though adding some weights to your yoga practice each week is a fantastic idea and combination—see part 3 for poses that include light weights.) Consistent practice of the various yoga poses builds strength and improves lean muscle mass. Through specific poses, you can concentrate on muscle groups that are underutilized or stretch out your overtrained and maxed-out muscles. Which muscles you need to strengthen and which you need to stretch and rest varies from sport to sport, so you can and should adapt your yoga practice to serve your specific athletic needs.

Physical strength will improve your endurance, surely something to be prized in sports such as cross-country or triathlons. But it's not just physical power that guides an athlete over the long haul; mental endurance is also key. Part 5 of this book gives you specific techniques for harnessing the power of your own mind. When you learn to tune in to your body and mind, everything can be a meditation—sports included. Yoga helps you learn how to pace yourself and focus on the moment, not on how long it's going to take to finish. It also develops a powerful foundation in your core, which is essentially the nucleus of your balance and movement.

Almost everything you do in life activates your core, and almost everything in yoga works on your core strength. When core stability is enhanced, it reinforces the supportive but otherwise underdeveloped muscles surrounding the more utilized muscles, creating a more balanced and optimal strength. Strong and stabilized core muscles in turn help with overall performance. Yoga helps strengthen all of the stabilizing muscles that are vital in protecting your joints and spine, among other things. People tend to miss these in other physical workouts, but your new yoga practice will bring them to life in order to enhance your body's overall functioning.

The core guides your balance, and your ability to balance through different movements can make or break your game. After all, balance is necessary whether you are shifting your feet closer together or farther apart, lowering your body to the earth, standing tall, jumping, swinging, or generating force. If your balance is on point, it gives you a solid ground to work from and helps maximize movements and prevent falls and injuries. Many of the poses in the sport-specific sections of this book work your core; I have also included a stand-alone section of core poses so that you will be sure to get some core engagement.

If you play tennis or golf, you know the value of range of motion. With improved joint and muscular flexibility—gained through yoga poses and stretching—your body's overall structure is improved, and your joint and muscle pliancy will foster greater range of motion or an increase in the performance latitude for a particular movement or series of movements. For example, a swimmer with supple shoulder and hip joints is able to capture and pull more water than a swimmer with a more limited range of motion. The result is more forward movement per stroke as well as enhanced muscular economy.

There is some dispute about the advisability of excessive stretching (for runners in particular), but I remain a huge advocate for it when it is done after a workout, finding that the more I work to maintain my flexibility (something that wanes with age), the less likely I am to suffer from an injury caused by an overuse of or a strain to the muscles.

Intense engagement in sports can be a huge strain on the body, and it is important to balance that with rest and recovery. Restorative yoga helps your body recover from any particular strain on the body, whether it's an injury or some other physical ailment. Yoga helps put athletes back together after a tough game or workout. By slowing down, you are allowing the body to heal and to tell you where it's tight and where future injuries may be brewing. Yoga also elongates all of the muscles that athletes spend so long contracting, so it is a great counteraction.

To quell the mind of your own mental chatter and of that around you is not easy, especially in a high-pressure moment. Yoga improves your control over that noise to create a center of focus and to promote serenity by silencing surrounding pressures, both internally and externally. When your mind learns to move with ease and stop forcing movements, you will prevent injuries and your body will open with your mind, increasing your flexibility, both mentally and physically.

the fundamentals of the yogafit approach

At YogaFit, we teach what we call "The Essence," which is comprised of seven areas of focus intended to help you be safe and comfortable on the mat. As much as adhering to the Essence components will help you on the yoga mat itself, I think you'll find that there are off-the-mat benefits too. As you embark on the sport-specific poses later in the book, keep these seven components in mind:

1. Breathe

Most often, we are just passively breathing, unaware and disconnected. The goal of taking specific time and focus to breathe, as in a yoga class, is to be deliberate or purposeful with your breath. Mindful breathing calls attention to your breath quality and how it affects your body and psyche; quick and shallow versus slow and deep, for example. YogaFit emphasizes deep diaphragmatic and controlled breath to improve your quality of breathing. In turn, as you improve, you not only reap the health benefits (such as reducing stress and symptoms triggered by stress), but you can improve oxygen efficiency.

Professional athletes are often tested for their CO_2 maximum. This test measures the amount of oxygen used by the whole body in a specified amount of time (milliliters of oxygen per minute per kilogram of body weight). This information helps to determine optimal training levels and performance potential. With specific training, and in order to improve performance, an athlete will gradually push their anaerobic threshold (or lactate threshold), which is the exercise intensity at which lactic acid starts to accumulate in the bloodstream. Full diaphragmatic breath helps to improve or maximize lung capacity, which aids in more efficient breathing, meaning the efficient use of oxygen that helps us reach optimal performance.

Oxygen fuels strength, movement, and cardiovascular endurance. Oxygen is the "what," the air you breathe in rest and during activity. Your CO_2 Max is the "how," a measurement of how your body utilizes the air you breathe in and converts it to energy. A strong and efficient CO_2 Max will enable you to perform longer while maximizing the oxygen you take in with each breath. Work on the breath ability, and your CO_2 measurement will improve.

Breath is also an innate tool to keep you calm and focused. When you inhale and let it go, it slows down the central and respiratory systems and helps shed nervous energy, which brings attention to the moment at hand. Think about it: Before taking the penalty shot, before leaping off the platform for the perfect dive, before preparing for that super lift, or whatever it may be, you can get "in the zone" with a long, deep breath. Look closely at professional athletes, and you'll see them do this as well. Intentional breathing gives you a specific moment of focus while relaxing your nervous system.

2. Feel

Tapping into your body and understanding what you *feel* could mean the difference between incurring and avoiding an injury. It all begins with breath, and once you are breathing more purposefully, you increase your body awareness. The purpose here is to notice what sensations the body experiences. Take your time and tune in—what do you feel right now and where? Do you feel calm or anxious, tense or relaxed? In yoga you want to feel something in every pose, no part of your body is just hanging out; instead, everything is energetically engaged.

3. Listen to your body

With this awareness of the sensations in the physical body, what are you to do? Everything you feel can be used as a guide. In her book *Your Body Speaks Your Mind*, Deb Shapiro explains that "every symptom is the way the body communicates; it is like a word or a message." You can use these messages to determine how far you can take your training or how long you can hold a pose in yoga. During your yoga practice, you can choose a pose option (whether it's modified or not) to incur more or less sensation according to your body's message. For instance, you may dial up the sensation for more intensity or dial it back for less. When on your yoga mat, choose according to what you truly need in the moment and in conjunction with your current training regimen. You may choose a more intense yoga practice in order to expand, grow, and progress into new abilities or accomplishments. Or you might choose a gentler yoga to take care of your aching body. This careful listening and choosing will reduce the chance of incurring an injury or aggravating an existing one.

4. Let go of competition

To tell an athlete to let go of competition is like telling a writer to not worry about words! As an athlete you are trained to compete—plain and simple. However, on the yoga mat, you have the chance to set the competition aside and live in that stress-free moment to focus on the poses. On the mat, there are no officials keeping score on pose execution, nor is there anyone around competing to hold a pose longer. It is you and your mat. Stepping onto the mat, athletes can embrace the moment and the yoga practice for themselves while focusing only on pose benefits and alignment.

5. Let go of judgment

This can be quite intense for an athlete. If you're a pro, you've got judges, fans, critics, and sponsors to worry about. As a weekend warrior, you've got your best friend, your spouse, or maybe even your children to impress or think about. Often there is an image to uphold or a level of performance to meet or exceed, and as a result you do what you can to achieve perfection in the spotlight, whether it's actual or imagined! You may even judge your peers, which is negative energy. However, on the mat and in the studio you can and should let go of judgment.

Practice your poses with a kind, compassionate heart, and use the positive mantras to encourage and appreciate yourself. Practicing yoga is a chance to encourage, not judge, yourself: "I am experiencing this pose with ease and confidence," or "Where I am at is where I am supposed to be." Be creative and be kind to yourself.

6. Let go of expectations

Letting go of expectations is about being open to possibility. *Anticipate everything, expect nothing.* You may come to your yoga mat with expectations that do not serve you. Instead, let go of any expectations of what the yoga experience will be and what your body can or will do. I love to say that "there is no perfect pose." However, there is a perfect pose for each body—the one that is necessary in each moment. Embrace the mat, be open and trust your body to do exactly what it can, which will make yoga far more enjoyable and beneficial.

Expectation usually keeps you attached to your desired outcome. If you hold on to an outcome you didn't expect, it disrupts your focus and sets you back, costing you valuable time in sports. Anticipation welcomes many ways to your desired outcome, such as a new personal record, a gold medal, or the Grey Cup. Like a soccer or hockey player anticipating the many possibilities of where the ball or puck will be next, anticipation keeps you ready and on your toes for the next possibility. NHL star Wayne Gretzky said, "A good player plays where the puck is. A great player plays where the puck is going to be."

7. Stay present in the moment

Yesterday is history, tomorrow is a mystery, today is a gift—that's why it's called the present. Have you heard those words before or something similar? It is true, the past has happened, it is history. You can learn from it, but you cannot change it. The future is beyond your reach, and it's a mystery what will happen. The present moment, on the other hand, is the only moment you really have any control or influence over, and for an athlete the present moment is crucial to effectively respond to what is happening.

So how do you stay in the present moment? On the mat, you simply bring yourself back to your breath—bringing The Essence full circle. As well as an innate tool to increase awareness of the physical body, breath is also your tool to be in the present moment. The body does not judge a breath it took yesterday or last week, and the body certainly is not going to worry about the next breath. The body is always present to the breath, so when you draw your attention to your breathing, you are drawn into the present moment.

PEP talks

In YogaFit, we practice giving PEP (Praise-Encourage-Praise) Feedback to others, and it is important to utilize this tool and apply this in your own internal dialogue when you're coaching yourself (for more on becoming your own coach, see Part 5). Through PEP Feedback you can build a safe dialogue with yourself and consider it a pat on the back or a moment of encouragement when you're feeling overwhelmed or frustrated.

PEP starts with a positive statement, then encourages you with a strong "help statement," followed by another positive statement. Most people find that understanding PEP as it pertains to how you speak to others—teammates and coaches, for starters—is the way to ease into communicating this way with *yourself*. Below are the PEP guidelines when speaking to others, which you can utilize to inspire your teammates and those around you.

Principles of Giving Constructive Feedback

- With an intention of being helpful, supportive, and encouraging, you ask permission before providing feedback. Some people do not take feedback well or are not open to it, so it is important to check to see if someone is in a mental space to listen.

- Focus first on the positive and then on how to improve. Deal only with a specific skill or technique that can be changed. For instance, your teammate is practicing free throws and you notice that their follow-through falls toward the left (and hence, so does their shot). First point out that they're doing a great job, then say how they can fine-tune their practice.

- Describe the skill or technique rather than evaluating it, and give them the why. Oftentimes relating a critique with a mapped-out reason why it works will help them understand *why* they should amend what they're doing. If you simply say, "Your wrist is going toward the left, center it more in your follow-through," they might not understand it. But if you say, "If you center your follow-through, the ball will follow!" then they will more likely comprehend what you're saying and why you're saying it.

- Relate objectively and specifically about what you have seen or observed. A good way to do this is to show them—do the free throw shot with a left-heavy follow-through, then do it again with it centered. Relay facts about skill or technique precisely and without exaggeration.

- Use "I" statements to accept responsibility for your own perceptions and emotions. Praise and encourage. Using "I" statements to accept personal responsibility means that you acknowledge your part in creating success or failure. "I did not fully swing the golf club, therefore the ball did not make the hole," or "I prepared myself via meditation and visualization so I was able to make that shot."

- Check to make sure that the recipient understood the message in the way it was intended. Avoid making the recipient "wrong" by wanting to be "right." Have your teammate show you before and after and then sit with them and watch while they work to improve.

- Avoid extreme or coercive language like "should," "always," and "never." These words can be negative and demanding. Instead of saying, "You should be shooting like this," say, "Your shot will improve if . . ."

Principles of Receiving Feedback

Now, if a teammate approaches you with feedback on your skill (and you are open to receiving it), here are some notes on how to accept it with an open mind.

- Listen openly, without excuses or judgment. Your teammate is giving feedback to help you improve, so hearing and absorbing what they have to say will ultimately improve your game. If you don't necessarily agree with the feedback, listen anyway and thank them graciously for taking the time to offer it.

- When you ask for feedback, be specific in describing the area of improvement. Rather than saying, "I need help with my chipping technique," say "Every time I chip the ball it goes too far. How do I tame my swing?"

- Let go of defensive reactions or temptations to rationalize the skill or technique at issue. This isn't easy to do. But if someone is trying to help you, try not to argue or give excuses for why you do a certain thing, because that reaction will only hinder your ability to listen, learn, and thrive.

• Summarize your understanding of the feedback. Repeat back what you learned so that your "teacher" will know that you heard what they had to say. Also, repeating will help you remember.

• Use "I" statements, share your thoughts and feelings about the feedback. Example: "I get it, thank you! I understand now why I don't do a full swing when chipping the ball."

Guidelines for Effective Feedback Exchange

When sharing mutual feedback, as you might do if you're sparring with another boxer or if you've been hitting the ball with another tennis player, it's important to ensure that both parties are willing to collaborate on feedback in order to up each other's game.

• Agree to be open and honest with each other with genuine care. For example, make sure you use nonthreatening body language, tone of voice, and word choice.

• Take notes! Writing down each other's feedback allows you to refer to it later. This is also a great opportunity to jot down questions about the feedback you are receiving. Listen attentively and ask questions.

• Phrase comments in positive terms. For example: "I think your swing can be improved by . . ." is the positive and more effective approach. "Your swing should never look like that" shuts the conversation down.

being your own coach

As much as offering feedback to others about *their* game, becoming your *own* coach will help you develop a positive you. Coaches observe their teams and athletes and recognize when something (or someone) is out of sync. It is their job to build up player confidence and strength; it's the way they will help a player or team get to a goal. I want you to do the same for yourself through an encouraging internal dialogue that leads you to success. When talking to yourself (it's OK, we all do it!), it is first key to recognize whether what you are saying is positive or negative. Both will impact you and your sport tremendously. Like your coach, you need to be supportive in your own growth, yet challenge yourself as well—you will be your best through positive yet firm reinforcement.

Your inner coach should be your best advocate, and it will help you achieve your goals. Below are a few guidelines on how to be your own coach:

- **Start a journal.** Journaling helps you to honor your thoughts and then to let them go. Oftentimes we bottle up our emotions and dwell on them, which then affects our focus and game. Journals do not judge those thoughts; rather, they allow you to expose those feelings that are weighing you down.

- **Practice gratitude.** Every day, write down three things that you are thankful for, whether it's about sports or not. If you're having a challenging day and you sit down to jot down three positive things, it will bring you back to center and remind you of the grace that surrounds you.

- **Write your goals and make a plan for each goal.** Making a goal tangibly visible with a plan on how to achieve it will help you realize it. Make a point to refer back to your plan once a week to see your progress.

- **List your fears and track your emotional responses**. Learn to observe your inner dialogue and how you respond to yourself in moments of stress. You want to be kind to yourself and avoid anger if something doesn't work out the way it should—if your calf muscle is too tight or if it's feeling weak during a game, yelling at your leg isn't going to help. Recognize what triggers your negative self-talk and develop positive alternatives.

- **Reevaluate and mark your progress daily**. Remember to check in on yourself to ensure that you are on track. Glance back at your goals you've written down. The only way to get back on track is to recognize that you are off it!

- **Don't be afraid to drop goals, but keep going on the ones that matter**. If a goal is getting in the way of your happiness or success in other, more achievable goals, it's OK to let go and try again at a different time.

- **Focus on your strengths and those things that are priorities.** It's easy to get lost in the small details that create minutiae in life. Daily, make a list of things you must achieve that day. Also list your overall goals for your game, sport, or physique. To learn more about your strengths, visit authentichappiness.org and take a strengths test. Neuroscience tells us to focus on where our strengths lie as opposed to those things that reside on the bottom of the strengths list (your weaknesses).

CHAPTER 2

Getting Ready for Yoga

So you're convinced that adding some yoga to your other athletic endeavors has great value and will up your game. Great—you're ready to get started! But first a few words that will help you understand the workings of the body and how it relates to your overall form and safety. The body is complex, and developing the knowledge of how it functions will help you listen to it and strengthen it. First, we will explore the importance of our core, balance, and posture and the role they play in our daily lives. Then I will teach you safe yoga practice to prepare you for your poses.

Core

Unfortunately, because a vast majority of us lead a rather sedentary lifestyle (all that sitting at desks and then sitting on our couches to recover!), we are a physically weak nation, especially in our cores. More than just the obvious abdominal muscles, your core encompasses all the muscles that are activated in your abdomen and torso.

Fitness pioneer Joseph Pilates referred to our core as the "powerhouse," the place where we generate power and control. Whatever *you* want to call it, the core is the epicenter of your body, and it supports all movements. Almost everything we do is reliant on core strength.

With power and control from your center, you will be able to move more efficiently and protect yourself from injury. From a strong and stable center you can channel your energy into your athletic performance. In sports, you ideally want to decrease reaction time to a point where core strength is automatic.

Higher levels of athletic training tend to look at strength and stability as the job not just of the core but of the whole torso, with all the parts forming a pillar from which our legs and arms move as an extension. If you have a weak torso and core, yoga will give you the opportunity to develop this part of your body with slow, intentional movements, building within you an awareness of your *entire* body and highlighting your weaker areas.

Core Performance and Athletes' Performance were (quite recently) two well-established, high-level athletic training organizations in the United States. They recently merged to become EXOS, an institution for sports ranging from the high school level all the way to pro sports. It was Athletes' Performance that wrote that "the dynamic relationship of the 3 parts of the pillar: scapulae, trunk and hips, create a stable base to move from." The entire trunk is a "power and control house"; my term "SPA Principles of Alignment" emphasizes this understanding.

With the exception of a few poses intended for complete relaxation, all yoga poses encourage core engagement and postural alignment. Specific poses such as Plank, Cobra, and Locust target the all-important core.

Balance

How many sports can you name that require some level of balance? Some sports—figure skating, hockey—may be a little more self-evident, while the need for balance in others—such as golf and basketball—doesn't seem too obvious.

Obvious or not, however, an athlete's ability to balance through different movements can mean success in *any* game. Think of this in terms of your center of gravity. Your body is in a constant relationship to the earth by means of height, mass, and girth. Your ability to balance is equal to your awareness of your center of gravity, especially while you are moving. If you don't have balance or an awareness of your center of gravity, you will fall over! The closer you are to the earth and the wider your base of support, the lower your center of gravity is and the easier it is to balance.

As you move your center of gravity farther away from the earth or narrow your base of support—opening your stance, jumping, reaching, swinging—the more you have to work to stay balanced. Your center of gravity will also change depending on the force your body generates outward and the amount of force that is exerted on the body. Your strength and control from your center allows you to move better when your center of gravity changes. Yoga postures take you through varying levels of stability based on these points.

In athleticism, good foot health is important in moving, balancing, and shifting your body during complex maneuvers. Your feet ground you. With a lot of your time spent in comfortable shoes, you don't necessarily use your foot musculature as much as you would if your feet were constantly bare. You wear shoes for good reason: they give you support in your activities and support from your environment. But they also disconnect you—quite literally—from the ground. Yoga gets you out of your shoes, barefoot on your mat, and more closely connected to the ground, a place where you can strengthen your feet and refine your balancing skills.

Posture

Without posture, core and balance training can only go so far. To complement your core training you must correct your posture and address any underlying issues there.

If your posture isn't aligned and strong, you are in danger of injury. Consider the ubiquitous back strain as an example. It is often a result of moving with unhealthy posture: reaching for something on the floor with a rounded spine, straightened legs, and loose or hanging abdominal muscles. While you sit, your lower body is supported by a chair, and your muscles atrophy because they aren't needed. Then you reach for something from standing, and your stabilizer muscles don't know what to do. The result: a back strain or more serious injury. Some people wear wide black elastic waistbands to "protect" the back—they are meant to give the back support while you are squatting or lifting—but we all actually have the musculature to do this without an elastic waistband! If you become reliant on artificial support, the muscles intended for the job take a leave of absence, causing more problems than before; you will naturally become weaker.

The body naturally avoids or protects itself from pain, whether physical or emotional, and often the compensation is to cringe or hunch over, both of which are inefficient or faulty movement patterns, and they interfere with healthy posture. In response to fear, the body instinctively moves into forward flexion of the spine to protect itself—you inadvertently hunch forward to protect yourself. Another example is anticipating the sense of falling, to which your body will react by clenching up in forward flexion. If the fear is unresolved, or not replaced with a more positive thought or emotion, then the body hangs on to it and the forward flexion persists. In sports, repetitive movements without correction may reinforce poor posture and stiffness as well.

Yoga reinforces what you already know about core strength, good posture, and efficient movement and calls us to refocus and move more deliberately while maintaining healthy posture. The poses in this book, with ideal execution and alignment, encourage the ideal posture through the engagement of the core. The yoga posture of Chair is essentially a squat, which is a movement seen in baseball, weight lifting, and football, right before the snap of the ball. With a strong core and posture, you can do a safe squat: You bend your knees to lower your body and center of gravity.

Position of the head is also important in healthy posture. Placed in alignment over and between your shoulders, your head is held in the most efficient stance, the position that requires the least amount of work or energy to support. It is supported with the strength of the whole body right underneath it. With your head out of position—as when you put your chin forward—you waste precious energy to support your head. Think about it: It takes more energy to hold in your hand a one-pound ball with your arm extended than it does to hold the same ball with your arm close to your body and your elbow tucked under the weight of the ball. Go ahead, try it. Now imagine if that ball was ten or eleven pounds, which is about the average weight of the human head. The point here is head position matters. In sports, where the head goes, the body follows.

safe yoga

Safe yoga is about developing a routine that is well rounded from start to finish and knowing what you are doing and why you are doing it—understanding the purpose and benefits of warming up and cooling down, for example, or how each sequence benefits your athletic focus. When you know the purpose of a particular pose, you are more equipped to decide whether it matches what your body needs. As you've learned, repetitive movements in sport may cause imbalances or asymmetries in the body, so understanding the demands of a sport or activity helps you to select poses to enhance performance or correct an imbalance.

Note that most yoga injuries occur from pushing the body too far and not properly prepping and cooling down. It is up to you to understand, listen to, and feel your body so you can grasp when you should stop and when you should continue. It is crucial to understand technique in order to avoid injury. In the yoga sequences featured in this book, transitions are smooth from pose to pose, with the focus on a full-body workout tailored for your sport. I offer modifications to suit the needs of various levels. Encourage yourself to take breaks; channel The Essence by letting go of expectations, judgment, and competition; and do not push yourself past your limits—you will know when you've reached your limit if you just listen and feel the signs your body is giving you.

In YogaFit, we express hatha yoga postures using our Seven Principles of Alignment, or "SPA," which are important to build a completely stable and strong center. The following seven principles are designed to support a safe yoga practice and create the optimal position for your body during movement and also while holding the poses. Remember these when doing your sport-specific poses, because SPA increases safety while simultaneously providing functional mechanical techniques that you can use in your sport. Remembering these principles is important in a healthy practice; they will help you modify your postures and transitions whenever it is necessary to accommodate your body.

1. **Establishing Base and Dynamic Tension:** *Ground yourself and pull energy from your midsection*—Root your feet into the earth and "stack" your joints—knees over ankles, hips over knees, feet hip-width apart. Employ your entire body by engaging and contracting your muscles to become stable in a pose.

2.   **Creating Core Stability:** *Use the muscles of the core*—The abdominals and glutes, that is, the muscles you use to sit down, should be employed to create core stability and to lengthen your body prior to moving into or holding poses for greater strength. This protects the joints, tendons, and ligaments.

3.   **Aligning the Spine:** *Stand up straight*—The spine is supported through core stabilization, and the head follows the movement of the spine. When moving into twists, flexion, or extension, start in natural spine (that is, standing straight).

4.   **Softening and Aligning Knees:** *Bend your knees*—In most poses, your knees stay in line with your ankles and point directly out over your toes. In general, your knees, when bent, will also remain in the same line as your hips. To avoid overstretching injuries, keep a slight bend in your knees at all times.

5.   **Relaxing Shoulders Back and Down:** *Pull your shoulders away from your ears*—When holding a pose, your shoulders should be drawn naturally back and down to help reduce tension in your neck and shoulders.

6.   **Hinging at the Hips:** *Bend at the waist*—When moving into and out of forward bends, hinge from the hips, using the natural pulley system of your hip joints and keeping a slight bend in the knees. I like to call this a "micro bend."

7.   **Shortening the Lever:** *Bend your knees and elbows*—When hip hinging, flexing, or extending your spine, keep your arms out to the side or alongside your body to reduce strain on the muscles of your lower back.

warming up, working out, and cooling down

At YogaFit, we teach yoga in "The Three Mountain Format": warmup, work, and cool-down. That's how I structure my classes, and it's how I recommend you structure your practice. Since yoga is a form of exercise that requires a combination of flexibility, strength, endurance, and coordination, we warm up at the beginning and save stretching for the end. In your warmups, you will prep your body by using large full-body moves (full range of motion) to activate and engage the muscles for complex or flexibility-oriented poses. Stretching, however, is reserved for your post-yoga workout to elongate muscles that were tightened and to relieve tension from ligaments and tendons that were overtaxed. Many people stretch as a pre-workout technique to reduce injury and prepare the muscles. However, scientific literature has not, to date, confirmed that flexibility exercises before the elevation of core body temperature are effective in reducing injury.

The muscular structure of the body provides movement and protection for the skeletal system. All actions in the body take place through the contraction or relaxation of muscles at the major joints of the body—shoulders, hips, and so on. Each of these joints has an inherent range of motion that starts at the bones and works its way through the muscles. In your specific sport, you use this joint/muscle pairing to throw a ball, run, kick, and swing.

Accommodating the various ranges of motion can be restricted if the soft tissues of the body, including the muscles, tendons (which attach muscle to bones), and ligaments (which connect bones) are not thriving. Certain factors can play into the tension of these workings, including stress, and working joints through a restricted range of motion is perceived as inflexibility.

The solution to increasing flexibility is to begin working the joints through the full range of motion in your warmups, which activates the muscles and, to a lesser degree, the tendons. Two essential properties of muscles that trigger muscle flexibility are elasticity and plasticity. The elastic properties of muscles allow them to return to their original state from a stretch. If this were not the case, muscles would lengthen continuously until they became so loose that no movement was possible!

The plasticity properties of muscles allow them to adapt to the continued stresses you endure. If muscles were not pliable, then you would not be able to strengthen or stretch them; they would just remain the same after each activity. Interestingly, both of these qualities become more evident when there is an elevation in core body temperature—better yet, muscles respond better if we work them when they are warm. Therefore, the most appropriate place to introduce deep stretching (and even strength and endurance work) is after an elevation in body temperature.

Once you have sufficiently elevated your core body temperature, you can then begin using movements that condition the body for greater strength, stretch, and flexibility. Your deepest flexibility stretches should occur near the end of your workout, when your body is at its warmest and elasticity and plasticity in your muscles are optimal.

finding your routine

Yoga and meditation/visualization will be most beneficial to you and your sport if you practice during the "off-season" as well. Supplement these practices into your weekly routines so that you can build, restore, and enhance your athletic abilities.

1. Pre-Season/Strength Training

Pre-season training is a delicate balance of overloading yourself to become stronger and injury prevention (this is where restorative yoga is important) to make sure that your strength-building efforts don't result in problems. This is a great time to "up your game" in terms of your yoga practice—to build core strength and enhance flexibility. While keeping to your regular training program, I suggest integrating your new meditation and yoga tools throughout.

Restorative Yoga: 2 times a week

Regular Yoga Practice: 2 times a week

Weight Training Yoga: 2 times a week

Core and Balance Yoga: 3 times a week

Daily Meditation

Daily Guided Imagery

Your regular training program

2. In-Season/Recovery Program

Daily recovery from in-season practice and injury recovery are very similar. Oftentimes, even in the daily practice training phase, you may experience a set of tight muscles that need extra attention or you may feel the need to work around a sore spot, just as we would with an injury. It may be difficult to work in a full yoga regimen on top of your regular training during the season, but starting off the week with your sport-specific yoga sequence will benefit you. Otherwise, restorative yoga is the perfect supplement to help your body balance out the intensity of your in-season schedule.

Depending on the feeling of your body—what's tight, sore, or injured—you can usually train around it, and I highly suggest that. Years ago, when I broke my wrist in a bike race, I went to the gym daily to weight-train and attached bands to my injured arm. At times I even had cables around my forearms; it may have looked very odd, but it worked. During my eight weeks of recovery, I lost very little muscle. When going through a recovery stage, meditation and guided imagery/visualization become even more important.

Restorative Yoga: 3 to 5 times a week

Yoga with Weights Modified: 1 to 2 times a week

Daily Meditation: 2 times a day

Daily Guided Imagery: 2 times a day, picturing perfect health

---
* If injured: Walking/stationary bike, if possible 2 times a week

---

3. Off-Season Maintenance

Many athletes take the off-season to rest and refresh; others end up getting deconditioned and gain weight. Since the latter will only hinder your ability to continue to grow in your athletic endeavors, it's crucial to stay in shape and use the flexibility of your time to explore and develop new skills. This is a great time to get a better handle on your yoga in every way.

Restorative Yoga: 2 times a week

Regular Yoga Practice: 2 to 4 times a week

Yoga with Weights: 2 to 4 times a week

Core and Balance Yoga: 2 to 4 times a week

Daily Meditation: 2 times a day

Daily Guided Imagery

Your regular off-season program

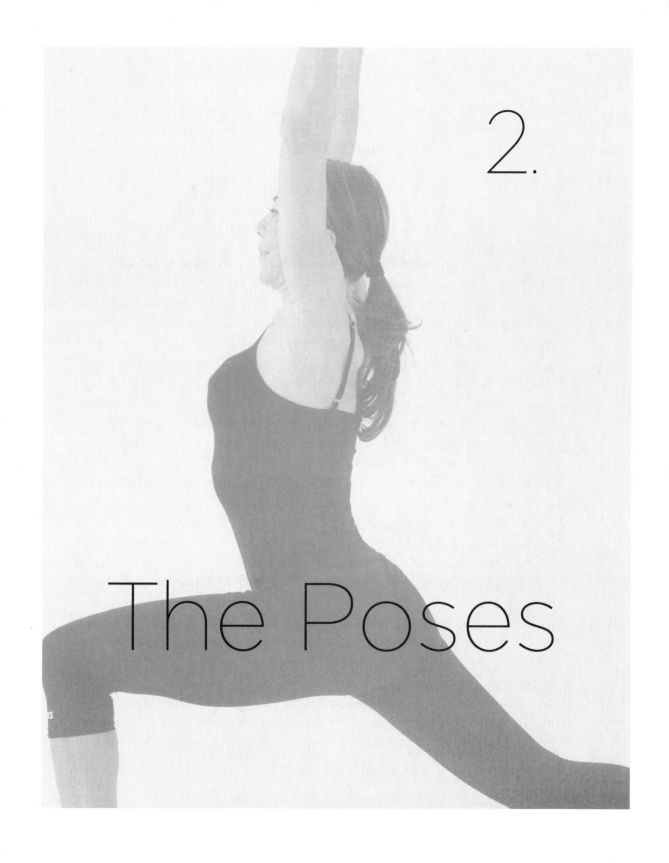

2.

The Poses

warmup flow sequences

As you know, yoga encompasses not only body engagement but also mind. Therefore, when you practice yoga, it's important to be in the moment and strengthen your concentration from pose to pose. Game-changing plays require a heightened level of focus and precision of movement; it is helpful for you, as an athlete, to leverage your yoga practice to visualize effective and successful performance. These poses give you the opportunity to delve into the intricacies of the athletic movements required for your sport at a slower, more methodical pace. During a yoga routine you can focus on both the physical and mental demands of your sport. When we slow down, continually make small adjustments in postures, and become aware (and engaged) in our body, thoughts, and breath, these skills will transfer to a refinement of our sports movement and a stronger kinesthetic or body awareness. When you incorporate these yoga routines into your training, you will ultimately experience increased power and precision of movement.

Any sport that requires single-side-dominant or repetitive movement that is not balanced will likely lead to muscle imbalances, therefore risking poor alignment and an increased potential for injury. The YogaFit postures can help train weak links, assist with imbalances, and ensure proper range of motion and mobility for enhanced performance.

The following are pose sequences that work well together and address the needs of your body to continue performing well in your sport. Every individual is different, and some poses may hit the spot while other poses have less of an impact. Get to know your body in your sport and in yoga. The poses listed address common areas and movements of the body as they relate to the sport and are intended for you to get the most out of your yoga practice. Pose selections will either complement or enhance movement demands of your sport or activity or offset the tightness that develops from repetitive movement. Tightness can often lead to restricted range of motion and therefore limit force production or strength when needed. My goal here is to keep your body moving in a variety of ways while paying attention to posture, balance, and core control.

This set of movements is intended to warm you up progressively and activate and stretch the whole body dynamically. Movement is generated from the hips and shoulders, using large muscle groups from light to moderate intensity. This series dynamically balances stretch and strength components of fitness to prepare the body for more intense work. It's a useful warmup segment for almost any sport.

Keep the sequences flowing from pose to pose, using your breath. Exhale when moving toward the ground and inhale as you lift up to the sky. As long as you breathe with movement, you will enhance the benefits of a warmup. It is not advantageous to hold stretches as a way to warm up. Imagine the muscles in your body as a piece of red licorice. When warm, the licorice is bendy and stretchy. If you eat your licorice from the fridge or even the freezer, you know that it is much less flexible. If you pull on it, it will snap. In fact, if you drop cold licorice, it might even shatter. For the body, this equates to injury, which we want to avoid, so reserve static stretches (holding) for post-exercise or sport. It is still common for people, especially weekend warriors, to start their sport or activity with deep stretches or stretch holds, which is not an effective warmup. Dynamic movement is the key—keep things moving.

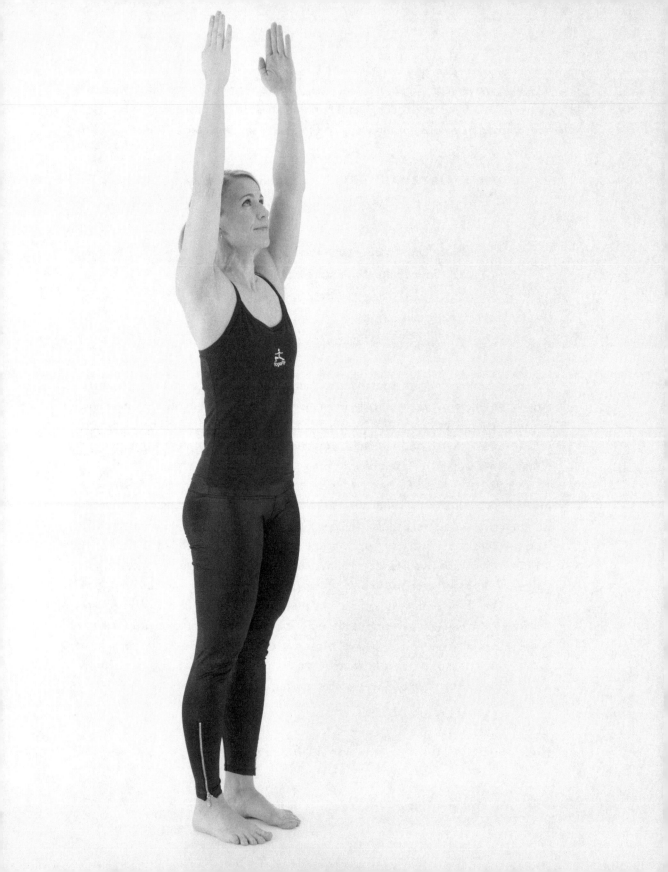

MOUNTAIN POSE with
BREATH AWARENESS

Benefit of the pose: Mountain Pose is a foundational pose. It is used often to begin practice and as a transition to other poses. Mountain is also your posture pose and a way for you to heighten your mind-body awareness. Having good posture and a strong mind-body connection will help you be alert and make your movements strong and efficient. It serves as a strong focal posture to begin a standing practice or to warm up with.

Getting into the pose: Stand with your feet at the top of your mat and observe your breath. From a strong connection to your mat, lift up through the arches of your feet. Activate your inner thighs and your pelvic floor and draw your belly in. Open your chest and soften your shoulders back and down from your ears. Lengthen your spine and continue to stand tall. Your arms can be at your sides or extended above your head.

Holding the pose: Create dynamic tension throughout your body, awakening all your muscles. Breathe more deeply with every breath—into your belly, your rib cage, and then your chest. Feel your body and notice your mind. With each breath, become more aware and more present.

CHAIR FLOW

Benefit of the pose: Chair to standing is beneficial for developing awareness in squat movement patterns—back position, placement of knees, and so on. Chair Pose builds strength in the hips, quads, abdominals, and upper torso. It trains you to use your core from a squat and back to standing while keeping a long neutral spine. It requires strength in the upper back muscles to stay lifted through the heart and avoid rounding your spine.

Getting into the pose: From Mountain, sit back, hinging your pelvis as if you are sitting down in a chair. Reach back with your tailbone and up through the crown of your head to lengthen your spine. Look down to see your toes in front of your knees.

Flowing this pose: Continue to inhale up to standing and then exhale back to Chair.

Modifications: If you find rounding in your lower back or shoulders, place your arms closer to your body or even rest your hands on your thighs for support and to reduce the load on your lower back.

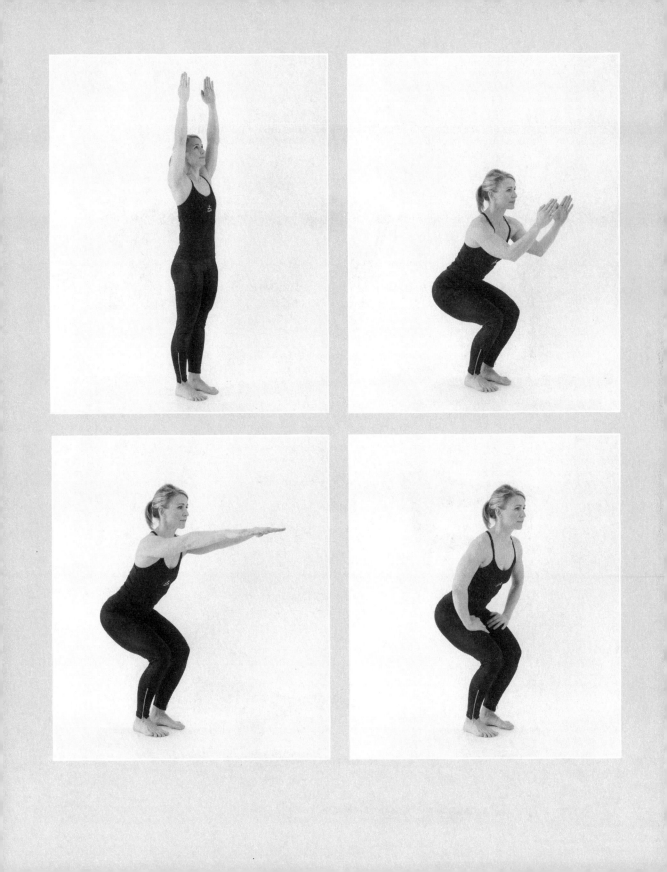

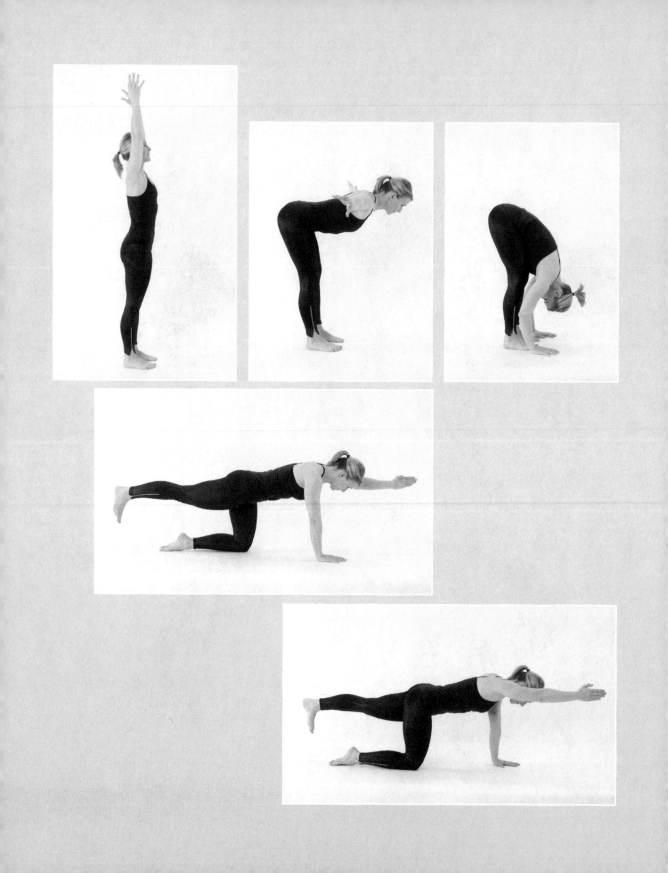

SWAN DIVE PRACTICE with SPINAL BALANCE FLOW

Benefit of the sequence: Swan Dive reinforces hip hinging with a neutral spine and establishes healthy movement patterns when going from standing to the floor and from the floor back to standing. Cat/Cow facilitates spinal mobility with flexion (rounding) and extension along your whole spine. Spinal Balance begins to activate your core for more stability and body awareness while you work through the movement of your arms and legs. All of these reinforce the always-important YogaFit SPA Principles, especially hip hinging, safe alignment of the spine, and core stability.

The flow: For all intents and purposes, when you flow you are moving with breath. You inhale by opening up your body and exhale by closing up your body. How you breathe and move is the buttress of dynamic movement and energy in your body.

Swan Dive Flow: Begin in Mountain and inhale your arms up. Exhale and bring your arms out to the side as you hinge at your hips into a fold. Bend your knees enough so that your belly can touch your thighs.

From the folded position, ensure that your core center is engaged, draw your shoulders back to open your chest. Inhale and reach your arms out to your sides, lifting your body back to Mountain Pose. Repeat 5–10 times.

Spinal Balance Flow: From all fours, work to lengthen your spine and stabilize your core center. With little or no movement in your torso, inhale and extend one arm and the opposite leg. Exhale and return your hand and knee to your mat. Inhale and switch sides, repeating 5–10 times per side.

DYNAMIC MULTI-MOVEMENTS with BREATH

Thus far, you've been doing dynamic (moving) warmup poses; the movements have been fairly basic, but you have been raising your body temperature and loosening up your muscles along the way. Next, I recommend a multi-movement segment. It is more complex and moves you in a variety of directions, increasing blood flow to more muscles, large and small.

The intention of this warmup is not to cultivate specific skills but to complement your existing training techniques and work toward a balanced spirit, mind, and body for optimal performance. Inhale deeply and exhale slowly with each of the following postures.

Downward Facing Dog: From all fours (where you were for Spinal Balance flow), reach your arms out in front of you and lift your hips to the sky, making an upside down V shape with your body.

Warrior Lunge: From Downward Facing Dog, step forward with your right foot into lunge. Keep your front knee over your ankle and lift your arms to the sky.

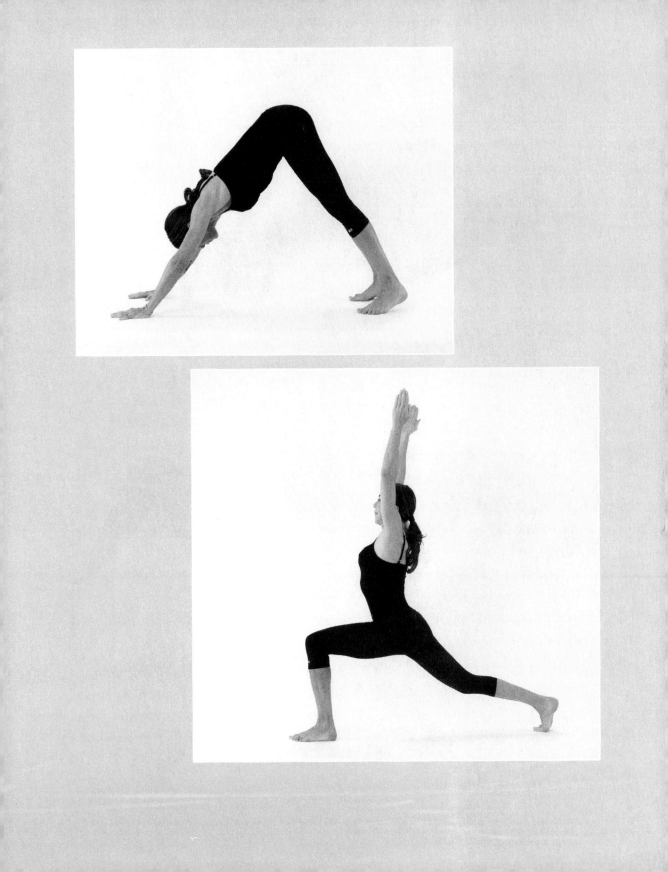

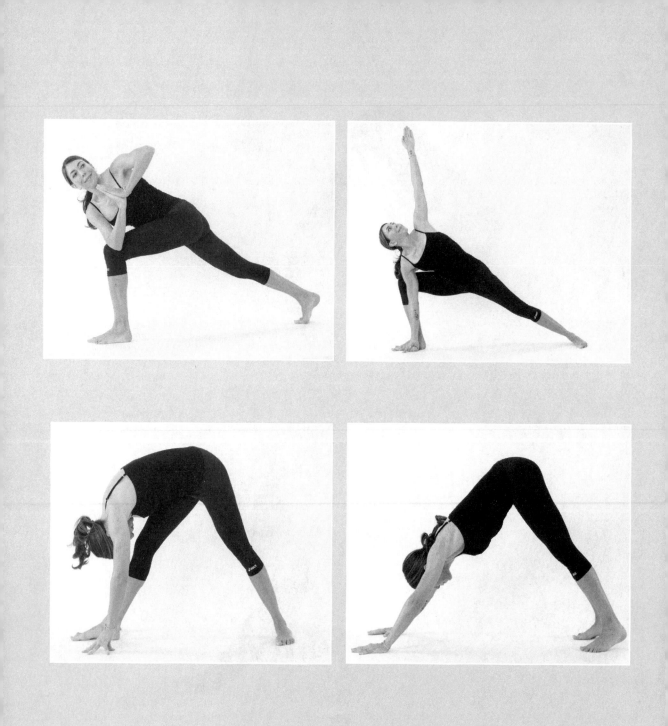

Twisting Lunge: From a Warrior Lunge, hinge forward over your right thigh. Twist from your belly, ribs, then your shoulders and bring your hands together, placing your upper left arm on the top of your right thigh. Option for stability: Place your left hand to the floor while you reach your right arm up to the sky.

Side Angle: From Twisting Lunge, release to the floor and place your right hand on the mat on the inside of your right foot or your forearm on your front thigh. Open your body to the side. Pivot your back foot to lower your heel to the floor and lift your left arm to the sky.

Pyramid: From Side Angle, turn to face the floor with your pelvis level. Straighten your front leg with a micro bend in your front knee.

Downward Facing Dog: From Pyramid, place your hands on the floor and step your right foot back. Lift your hips to Downward Facing Dog.

- Repeat the sequence with the left leg forward.
- Repeat the whole sequence 5–6 times per side.
- Progress to flow this sequence with a single inhale and exhale for each pose.

DOWNWARD FACING
DOG FLOW (4 POSITIONS)

Benefits of Downward Facing Dog: This pose opens you across your chest and offers space for the diaphragm and abdomen to breathe fully. It opens the front of your shoulders while building shoulder strength. It stretches the whole back of your body, including your calves, hamstrings, glutes, and major back muscles. This pose releases tension in the body and, through the inversion effect, aids blood flow to your brain. It creates a sense of alertness to prepare you for what comes next. With regular practice this pose can be very restful.

Benefit of this flow: This flow encourages you to feel each point of alignment in Downward Facing Dog while dynamically stretching key muscles for power, such as calves, quads, hamstrings, and glutes. As a dynamic stretch, it may help to loosen muscle fibers.

Flowing this sequence:

Inhale onto the tips of your toes.

Exhale and deeply bend your knees and hinge your hips (almost to Child's Pose).

Inhale and reach your tailbone to the sky to lengthen your spine.

Exhale and press your heels to the floor and lengthen your legs.

Modifications: If you have a hard time keeping your spine from rounding, bend your knees to keep your hips hinged and your spine long. To relieve tension in your wrists, come down onto your forearms with your elbows shoulder-width apart. Child's Pose is also an option for a rest at any time.

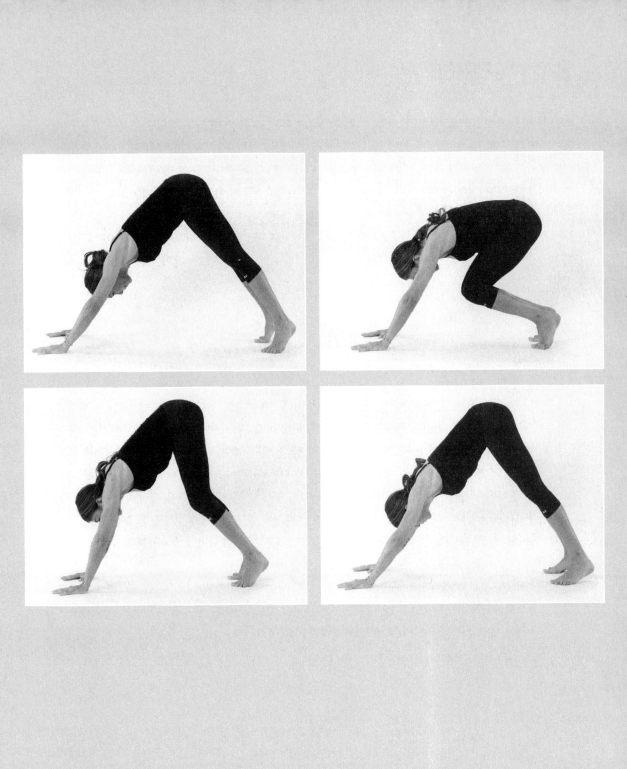

HALF SERIES

The Half Series integrates the upper body for a complete warmup. Right from the previously mentioned Downward Facing Dog Flow, you can execute the Half Series as an extension of your warmup. It is a great opportunity to exercise your cardiovascular system as well. Demanding more from the upper body than the standing postures in yoga, the Half Series is useful for athletes whose sport is lower body–dominant, such as soccer. In addition to a warmup, this series is a good bridge between standing poses to create upper body strength and to give your legs a break. Use the Half Series between each standing pose for extra work.

Half Series:

Downward Facing Dog—Plank—Crocodile—
Upward Facing Dog—Downward Facing Dog

From Child's Pose, exhale and lift your hips into Downward Facing Dog. Inhale, lower your hips, and shift forward into Plank, aligning your shoulders directly over your wrists. Ensure that your hips are in line with your heels and shoulders. Exhale and lower down to Crocodile with your arms tucked against your rib cage and your shoulders and elbows equal distance from the floor. Flip your feet and inhale, pulling forward into Upward Facing Dog. Exhale and lift your hips to the sky, go back into Downward Facing Dog. Repeat from Downward Facing Dog 3–5 times.

Modifications: As well as you can, keep the intensity up with the Half Series for a more athletic flow. However, if you require less intensity, move through the series on your knees using the Kneeling Half Series on page 42.

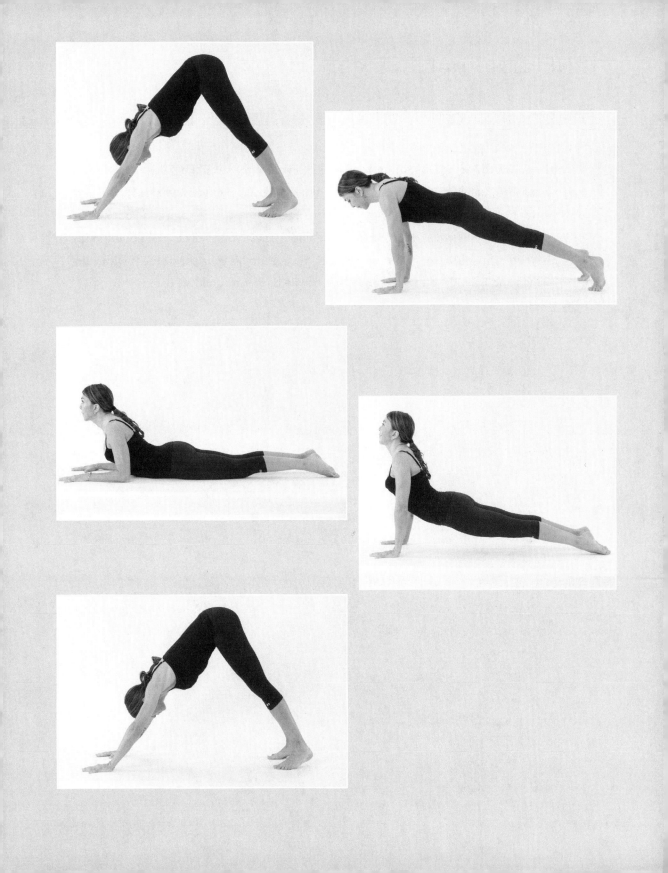

KNEELING HALF SERIES

Child's Pose—Kneeling Plank—Kneeling Crocodile—Cobra—Child's Pose

From Downward Facing Dog, bring your knees to your mat into Child's Pose. Inhale forward into Kneeling Plank with your shoulders directly over your wrists. Exhale and lower to Kneeling Crocodile with your arms tucked to your rib cage and your shoulders and elbows equal distance from the floor. Lower your belly to the floor and inhale up into Cobra using your upper back muscles to lift your chest. Press with your hands and lift with your core center and exhale back into Child's Pose.

SPORT-SPECIFIC POSES

Baseball/Softball

With throwing and swinging movements originating from the same side each time, baseball and softball tend to build a dominant side of the body. Even if you're ambidextrous, you will likely have a favored side. Necessarily, you are bound to have imbalances in your strength and range of motion that leave you at a slight disadvantage on your weak side and also vulnerable to injury on that side.

Baseball is a sport of multiple movement patterns, which include throwing, hitting, running, and gaining position for catching the ball. A baseball player is required to work at multiple tempos as well, responding with speed and accuracy to the demands of the game. To achieve the most precise and powerful movement, a perfect point of balance is required in order to accomplish quick direction change, powerful first-step quickness, and mobility.

The requirements of the sport can also be viewed from positional perspectives. Many movement patterns are similar, but some are very specific to the position played. A catcher is required to squat for long periods of time, while also needing to stand quickly from a deep squat position to execute a powerful and accurate throw to any given base. A pitcher stands on the mound, harnessing energy to produce powerful and accurate pitches. Range of motion for a pitcher is important; muscles need to be both strong and elastic enough to produce a forceful throw that is both precise and fast. In addition, breath control, which you learn in yoga, combined with fine motor skills, enables a pitcher to fine-tune his or her range of pitches and techniques—a fastball, slider, or knuckleball. Such pitches are achieved through controlled skill and by producing power through whole-body movement.

When a batter prepares for an at-bat, he or she needs to get in the zone, gather his or her thoughts, and focus. Once mentally prepared and up at the plate, stability and commanding rotational power combine with hand-eye coordination to yield success. If you're playing the infield or outfield, you are required to have a fast reaction time with the ability to move smoothly and quickly. Oftentimes, you might even stretch the entire body to grab for a ball. Your yoga practice will hone these important attributes.

As in any sport, the mental capacity to relax, focus, react, and execute game-changing plays in a matter of seconds (sometimes milliseconds) creates high demands on the body. Proper recovery and rejuvenation are an integral part of longevity in baseball, and with the significant likelihood of acute injuries due to spontaneous reaction in a play, it is crucial to develop a strong, balanced, and supple body.

STANDING STRADDLE SPLITS

Benefit of the pose: Standing Straddle Splits stretch your inner thighs and hamstrings.

Getting into the pose: From a standing position, step back with one foot and turn to face the long edge of your mat. Adjust your feet so that both feet are pointing forward, toes slightly turned in to align the outside of your foot with the short edge of your mat.

Holding the pose: Inhale and lengthen your spine, exhale and fold deeper into the pose.

Modifications: Move your feet apart to get closer to the floor. If your head easily reaches the floor, move your feet closer in and work to reach your head to your mat, developing strength in the hips and spine. For more support, place your hands on your thighs or a block to ease tension in your lower back.

Option to revolve: Place one hand directly under your gaze on the floor or a block. Lengthen your spine in a neutral position and twist first from your navel, then your chest, then your shoulders. The other hand may rest on your lower back or reach up to the sky.

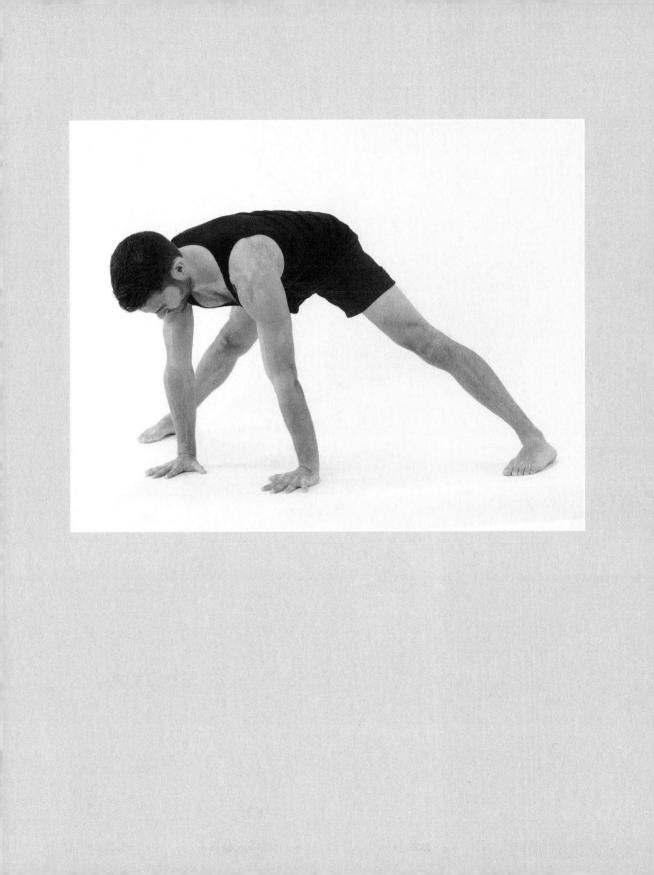

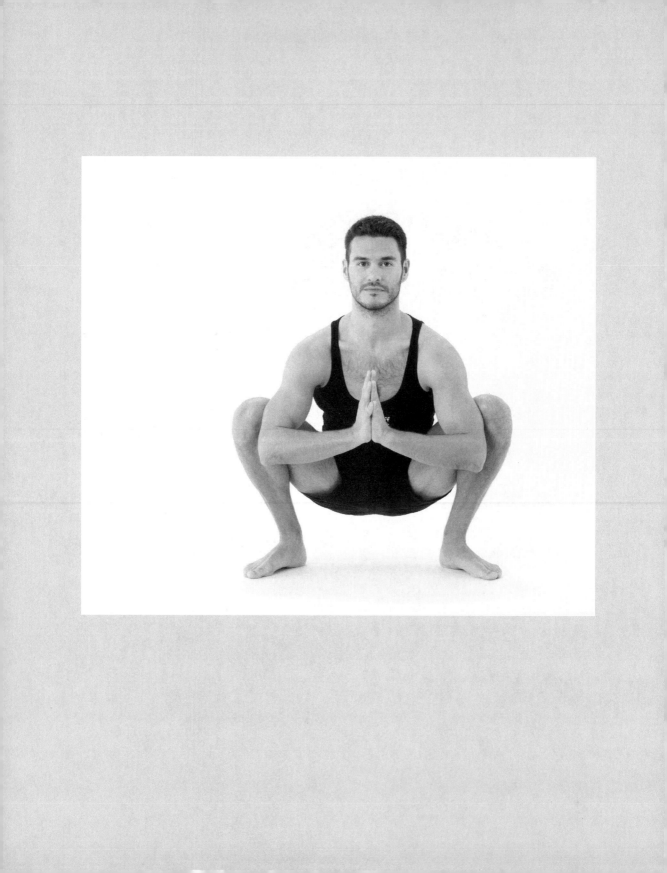

GARLAND

Benefit of the pose: Essentially a deep squat, Garland strengthens your hips, thighs, and upper back muscles. It is very functional for getting up and down from the floor and increases your range of motion in your hips while releasing tension.

Getting into the pose: From Standing Straddle Splits, shuffle your feet inward to a comfortable position. Place your hands or forearms on your thighs and lower your hips toward the floor, keeping a neutral spine. Adjust your foot position as necessary to keep your whole foot on the floor. As you lower your hips below the knees, keep your upper body raised, heart open.

Holding the pose: Work your upper back to stay lifted in your spine. Shift your weight from foot to foot and adjust their position so that your feet, ankles, and calves are comfortable. Stay extended in the upper spine.

Modifications: If you tend to round your back, keep your pelvis a little higher (level with your knees) and your hands on your thighs. Gradually work to lower your pelvis a little more. Roll or fold a mat to form a wedge and place it under your heels so that your feet and calves may relax.

DOWNWARD FACING DOG

Benefit of the pose: This pose opens you across your chest and helps you breathe fully through your abdomen. It opens the front of your shoulders while building shoulder strength. It stretches the whole back of your body, including calves, hamstrings, glutes, and major back muscles. This pose releases tension in the body and, through the inversion effect, aids blood flow to your brain. It creates a sense of alertness to prepare you for what comes next. With regular practice this pose can also be very restful.

Getting into the pose: From Child's Pose, tuck your toes under and reach your arms ahead. Press into your toes and spread your fingers wide while you lift your hips to the sky. Make an inverted V shape with your body.

Holding the pose: Inhale to reach your tailbone up and lengthen your spine. Exhale to bring your chest and belly toward your thighs.

Modifications: If you have a hard time keeping your spine from rounding, bend your knees to keep your hips hinged and your spine long. To relieve tension in your wrists, come down onto the forearms with your elbows shoulder-width apart. Child's Pose is also an option for a rest at any time.

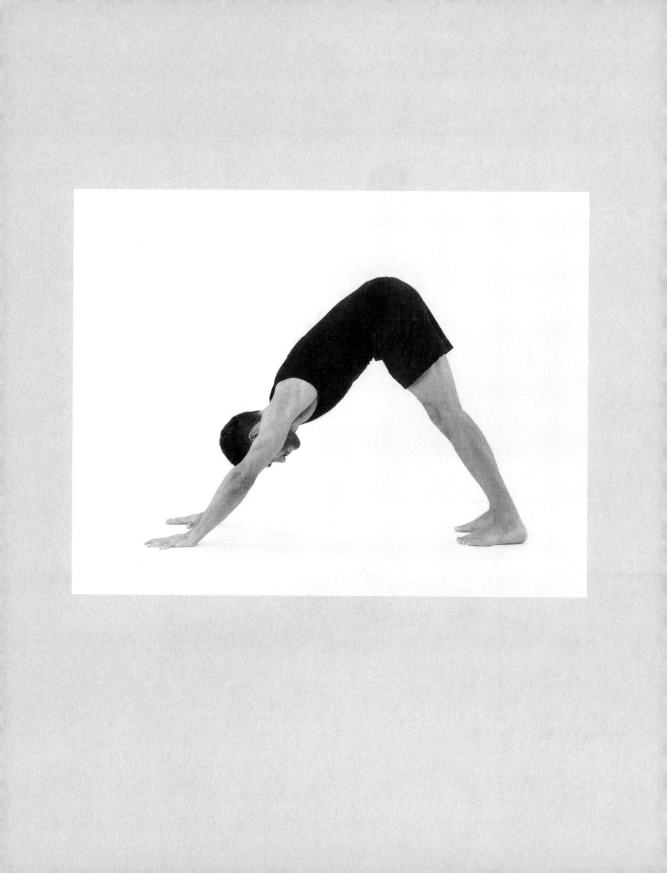

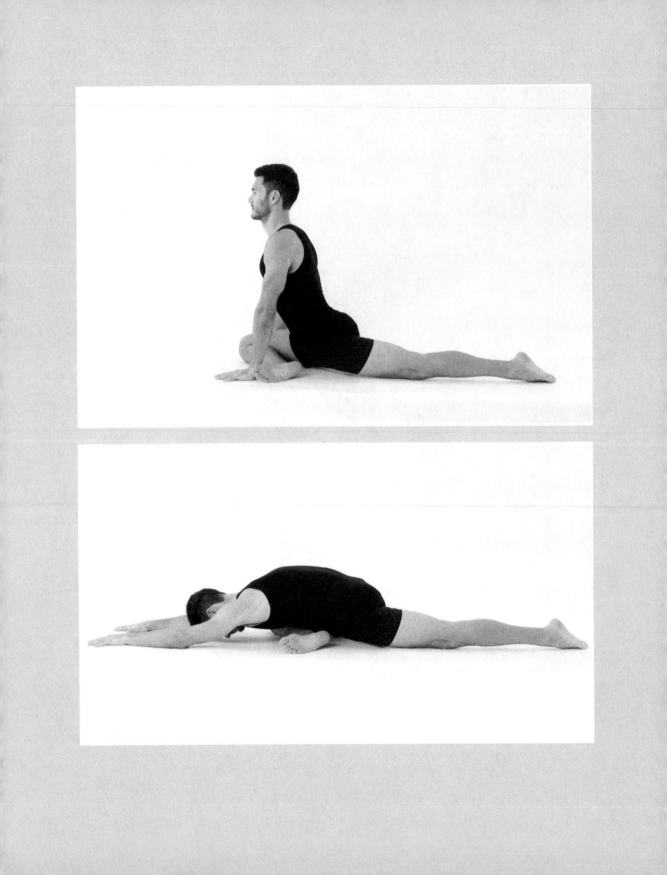

PIGEON

Benefit of the pose: Great for releasing tension and stress, Pigeon stretches the deep glute muscles in the back of the hips. It also helps to stretch the band of muscle that runs down the outside of the thigh from the hip to the knee that gets tight with a lot of running (IT Band).

Getting into the pose: From Downward Facing Dog, bring one leg forward to the floor with your knee bent and your foot flexed. Stay lifted enough to keep your pelvis level.

Holding the pose: Release your upper body down to the floor and rest your forehead on your hands or stacked fists.

Modifications: To make this pose more restorative, lie on your back with your knees bent and your feet on the floor. Lift one leg and place your foot on your other thigh for support. Reach to hold the supporting leg behind the knee and draw your leg in toward your chest. If your range of motion allows, Standing Pigeon from Chair Pose is another option. Bring one ankle to the top of the opposite thigh with your foot flexed and sit back into Chair Pose.

LOCUST

Benefit of the pose: This pose strengthens the entire back of the body, including your hamstrings, glutes, back extensors, upper back, and rear shoulder muscles. It also prepares you for more intense back work in poses like Bow and Camel.

Getting into the pose: Lie facedown and turn one cheek to the floor with your arms to your sides. Reach with your toes and activate your inner thighs and core center, lifting your belly button toward your spine. Reach your shoulder blades toward your spine, lifting your chest and shoulders away from your mat, and let your head follow. Keep your palms facing inward and reach your fingers toward your feet.

Holding the pose: Maintain a good connection through your core center to protect your lower back. Imagine that you are stretched like a hammock and continue to reach your toes and head away, spreading the work throughout your body.

Modifications: For less sensation, bring your hands back to the floor under your shoulders, as in Cobra, for more support. For more sensation, lift your legs away from the floor, keeping your feet together.

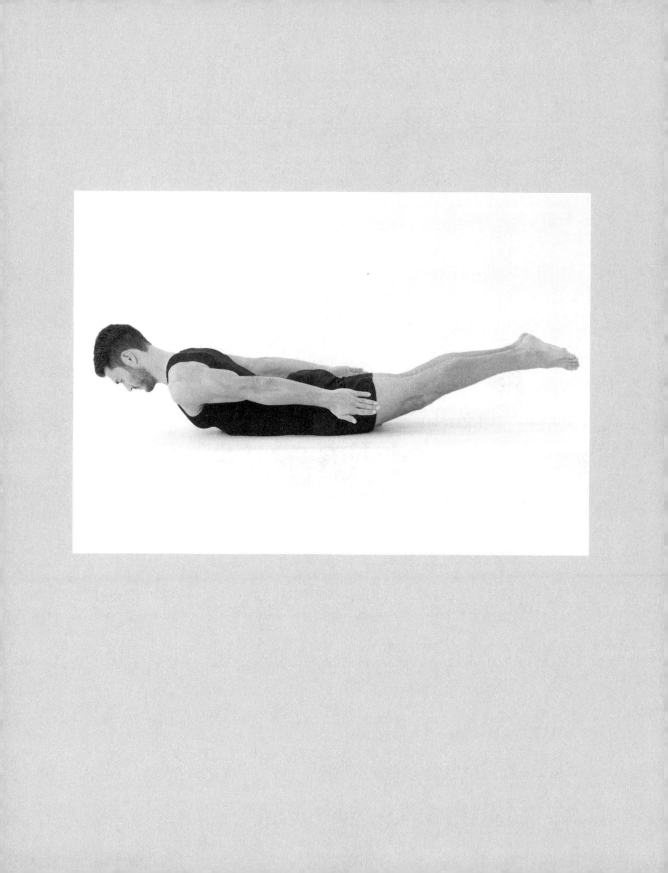

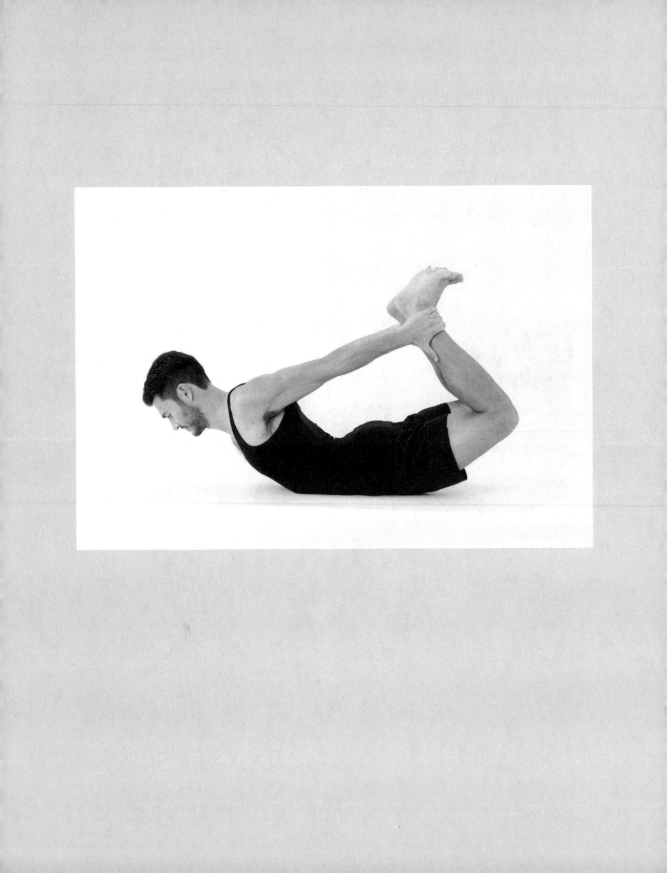

BOW

Benefit of the pose: Bow opens up the whole front side of the body—quads, hip flexors, abdominals, chest, and shoulders—while strengthening the entire back side of the body, including your hamstrings, glutes, back extensors, and upper back. Performed with intense levels of exertion, it helps the body to release tension and pent-up energy. This pose is great for offsetting excessive amounts of forward flexion (rounding of the spine and shoulders).

Getting into the pose: Lie on your belly and open your shoulders to reach behind to your ankles. Flex your feet and draw your thighs inward. Press your ankles into your hands and hold your ankles firmly. Engage your core center and lift away from the body.

Holding the pose: Keep a strong core center and continue to lift through the crown of your head and press your ankles into your hands.

Modifications: If you have difficulty getting both hands to your ankles, use Half Bow, which is performed one side at a time. Place one arm in front of you bent at the elbow. Use your hand and forearm across your mat for support and reach your other hand to the ankle on the same side. Another option is to place a strap around your ankle and hold on to the strap.

Basketball/Volleyball

In volleyball and basketball, skill is required to jump high and be quick on your feet to react to a play. In both sports, squatting prepares you to generate power for a jump or a fast move, and a semi-squat, much like Chair Pose, serves as a ready or guarding position. The following poses support you to build awareness in your movement as well as develop strength in opposing areas of the body for balance.

In both sports, plays are made while in the air, so a strong core (gained through Plank and other poses) will provide a strong foundation for power hits and precise shots when your feet are not on the ground. In these instances, stability must be achieved in midair. Play at the net for a volleyball player requires lateral mobility, balance, and vertical jumping skill. This also happens in basketball when guarding an opponent, squatting low and moving laterally to then jump vertically to block a shot.

Range of motion enables many players to "play bigger," cover more net or more space in a defensive position. This, along with breath control, can enhance your ability to manage your movement, recovery, and exertion in the game.

Some of these games may also demand play on one foot, increasing your balance requirements. In the yoga pose Warrior III, single leg balance is promoted and can be achieved through arm movement or knee bends. You might find it shocking how much work is required to just hold still. This can be a welcome challenge for you as an athlete: You'll get to focus more on muscular control specifically for balance as opposed to the larger gross motor skills like speed, power, and strength, which you are typically accustomed to.

DOWNWARD FACING DOG FLOW (4 POSITIONS)

Benefits of Downward Facing Dog: This pose opens you across your chest and helps you breathe fully through your abdomen. It opens the front of your shoulders while building shoulder strength. It stretches the whole back of your body, including your calves, hamstrings, glutes, and major back muscles. This pose releases tension in the body and, through the inversion effect, aids blood flow to your brain. It creates a sense of alertness to prepare you for what comes next. With regular practice, this pose can be very restful.

Benefit of this flow: This flow encourages you to feel each point of alignment in Downward Facing Dog while dynamically stretching key muscles for power such as calves, hamstrings, and glutes.

Flowing this sequence:

Inhale onto the tips of your toes.

Exhale and deeply bend your knees and hinge your hip
(almost to Child's Pose).

Inhale and reach your tailbone to the sky to lengthen your
spine.

Exhale and press your heels to the floor and
lengthen your legs.

Modifications: If you have a hard time keeping your spine from rounding, bend your knees to keep your hips hinged and your spine long. To relieve tension in the wrists, come down onto the forearms with your elbows shoulder-width apart. Child's Pose is also an option for a rest at any time.

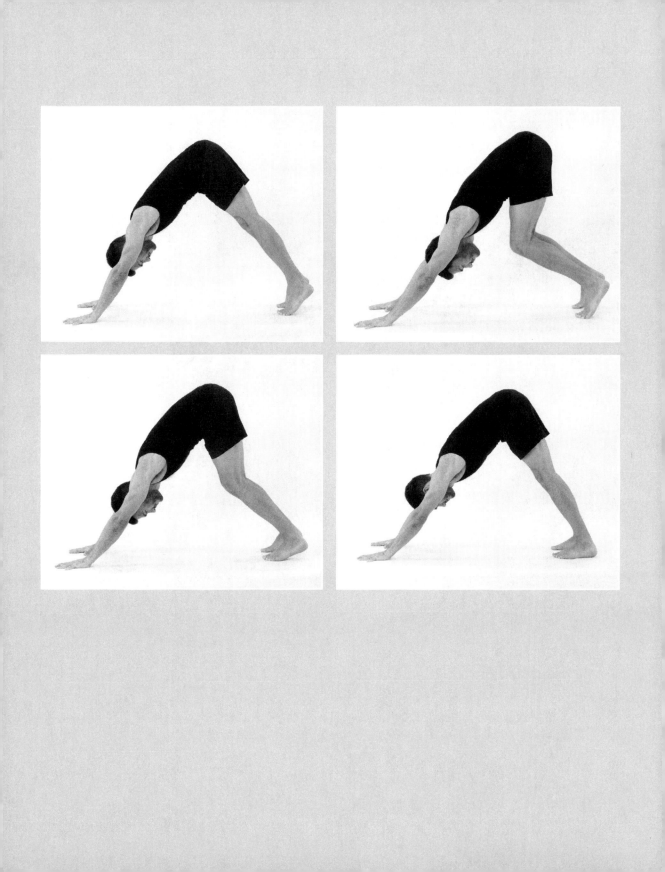

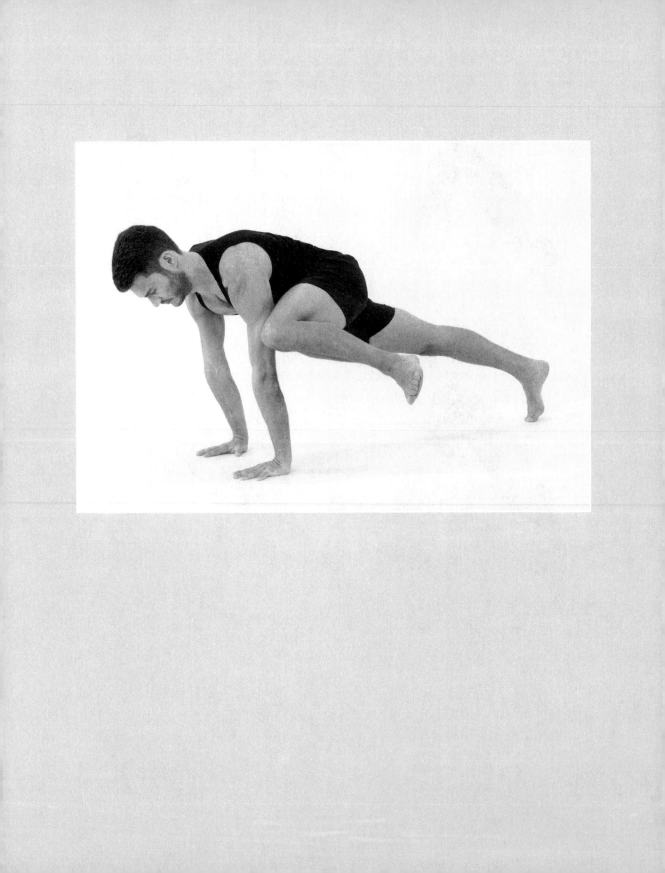

PLANK with KNEE to ELBOW

Benefit of the pose: This pose challenges your whole torso strength and stability from hips, core, and shoulders.

Getting into the pose: From Downward Facing Dog, shift forward so that your shoulders are directly over your wrists. Bend the knee of one leg slowly, moving it under your body so that your knee reaches your elbow on the same side.

Holding the pose: Lift with your core center and press away from your mat. Keep your gaze ahead and find stability in this pose. You may choose to flow in and out of this pose and back to Downward Facing Dog with your breath; inhale and shift forward to Plank and, as you exhale, shift back to Downward Facing Dog.

Modifications: Flowing may allow you time to work up to the strength required for the hold, gradually increasing the length of time you hold.

WARRIOR III

Benefit of the pose: Warrior III incorporates strength and balance. It strengthens your hamstrings, glutes, back extensors, hip, and core stabilizers. It also increases focus and concentration. This pose is effective to develop strength and control in movements such as diving and reaching for the ball.

Getting into the pose: From a standing position, extend one leg back and place your hands on your pelvis to start. Keep your pelvis facing forward and hinge forward from the hip of your standing leg and keep a micro bend in the knee. While you dip your upper body down, extend your back leg further up to make a straight line from your heel to the crown of your head and fingertips.

Holding the pose: Reach your arms forward or to the sides and extend your spine to work the core center and strengthen your back muscles. Reach your raised leg away to work the glutes and hamstrings, keeping your hips, knees, and toes pointing to the floor. Stand tall on your supporting leg.

Modifications: For less load on your lower back, bring your arms closer to your body and place your hands together at your heart. To offer support and prevent fatigue, place your hands on your thigh.

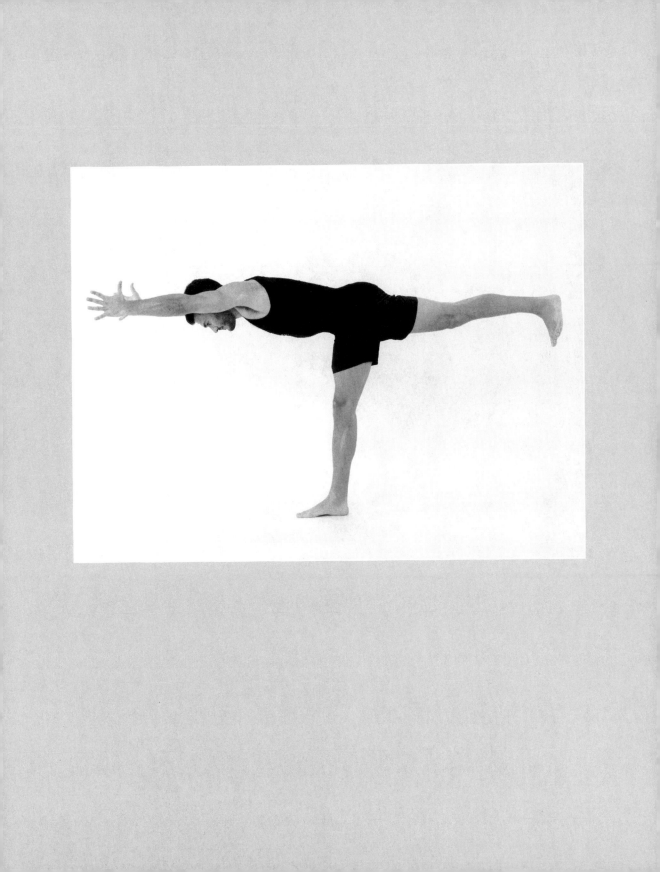

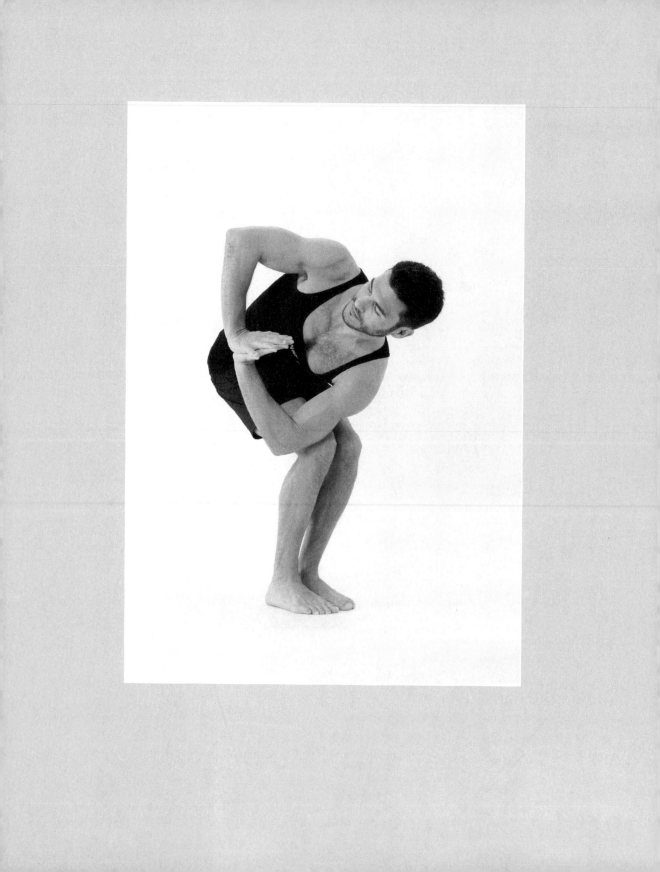

REVOLVING CHAIR

Benefit of the pose: Much like Chair, this strengthens your hips, quads, and upper torso. It also strengthens your obliques and stretches your lower back. The twist invigorates your torso muscles, stimulates conductivity of your sensory nerves, and massages your internal organs. Revolving Chair also trains torso rotation with open chest and shoulders, which you need for an effective tennis or golf swing.

Getting into the pose: From a standing position, bring your feet and legs together and sit back into Chair Pose (see page 30) with your hands together at your heart. From Chair, keep your legs and feet together and twist first from your navel, then your chest, then your shoulders. Once in the twist, you may also open up your arms and reach to the floor and sky.

Holding the pose: Breathe in to lengthen your spine and breathe out to rotate further. Keep your knees level with each other. As you reach your arm to the sky, pull the shoulder blade on the same side toward your spine to open your chest. Engage your core center to support your spine.

Modifications: For less sensation and more support, bring the arm on the side you are twisting toward onto your lower back. Gently reach across and place your other hand on the opposite thigh.

GARLAND

Benefit of the pose: Essentially a deep squat, Garland strengthens your hips, thighs, and upper back muscles. It is very functional for getting up and down from the floor and increases your range of motion in your hips while releasing tension.

Getting into the pose: From Standing Straddle Splits, shuffle your feet inward to a comfortable position. Place your hands or forearms on your thighs and lower your hips toward the floor, keeping a neutral spine. Adjust your foot position as necessary to keep your whole foot on the floor. As you lower your hips below the knees, keep your upper body raised, heart open.

Holding the pose: Work your upper back to stay lifted in your spine. Shift your weight from foot to foot and adjust their position so that your feet, ankles, and calves are comfortable. Stay extended in the upper spine.

Modifications: If you tend to round your back, keep your pelvis a little higher (level with your knees) and your hands on your thighs. Gradually work to lower your pelvis a little more. Roll or fold a mat to form a wedge and place it under your heels so that your feet and calves may relax.

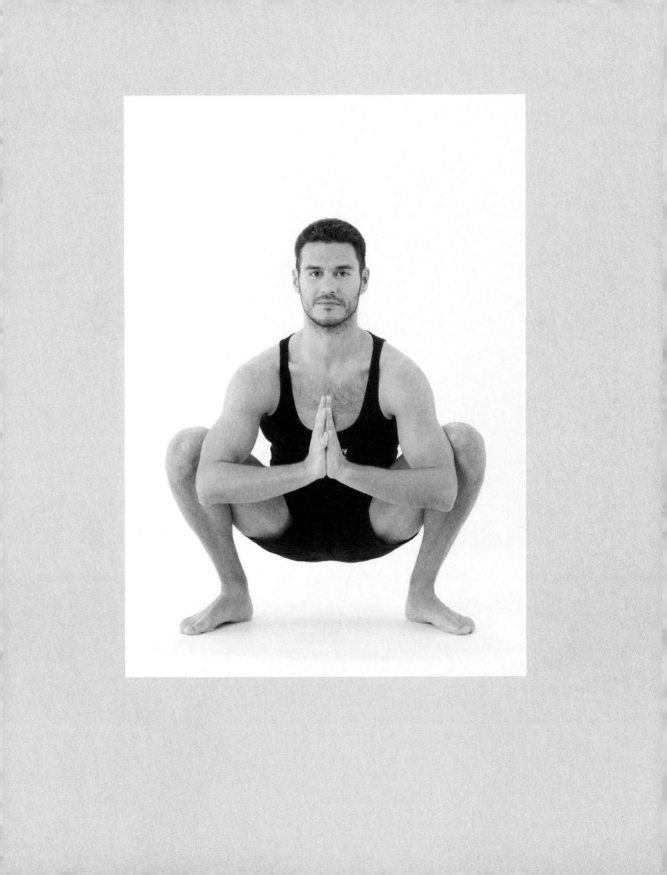

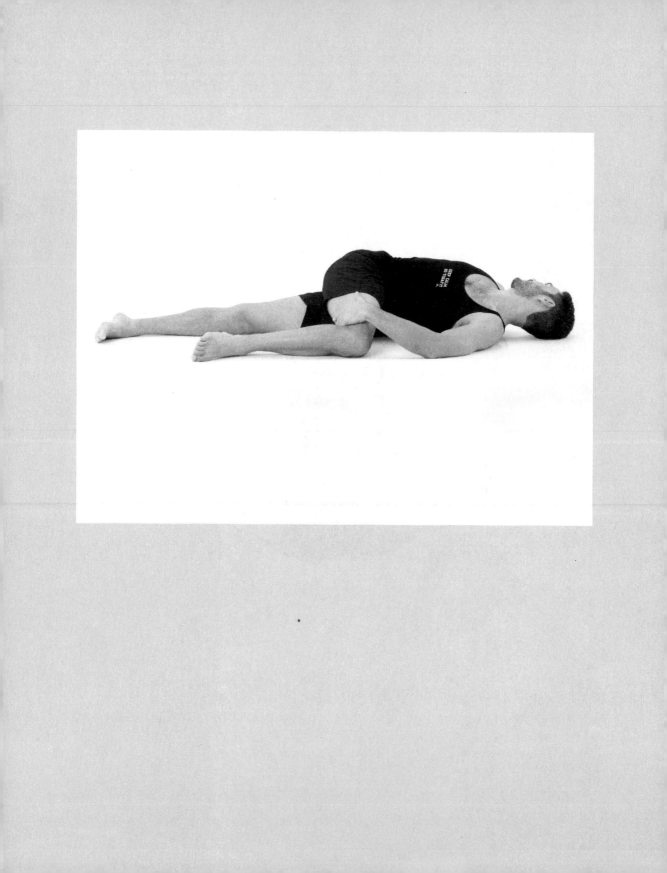

SUPINE SPINAL TWIST

Benefit of the pose: This pose will help you stretch out your lower back and open up your thoracic spine. From a lying position you can lengthen your spine with ease because you don't need to work against gravity. The twist invigorates your torso muscles, stimulates conductivity of your sensory nerves, and massages your internal organs.

Getting into the pose: Lie on the mat on your back and bring your right knee to a bent position with your foot on the floor beside your left leg. Press into your foot and lift your pelvis up enough to shift your pelvis to the right and then rest it on the floor. Keep your right shoulder on the mat and use your left hand to gently draw your right knee over your left and toward the floor.

Holding the pose: Keep both shoulders placed on the mat and look over your left shoulder to maximize the benefit of the twist. Practice releasing toward the floor with every exhale, then switch sides.

Modifications: From a side-lying position, rotate your upper body open, keeping your hips facing the side. Place a block or two under your right knee or a rolled-up mat lengthwise behind you for support. If you have any disc injuries, this may aggravate the injury. In this case, start with both knees bent and allow both legs to go to one side.

Bodybuilding/Weight Lifting

Bodybuilders and weight lifters need to manage a lot of weight right above the torso. Therefore, it is incredibly important to have impeccable shoulder and hip stability when practicing this sport. Without this stability you are an injury waiting to happen. Most often, power lifters train with total body movement. However, a bodybuilder, at least traditionally, focuses on defining specific and isolated muscles. However you are training for strength and muscle definition, your movement is likely to become rigid and your body will feel stiff. Unintentionally, you may leave important muscles untrained and weak, which can result in injury. Yoga moves the body with fluid total body movements that lengthen the muscles while also creating strength and body awareness. Static or stationary holds in yoga poses can sometimes mimic the poses that bodybuilders hold and concentrate on a specific muscle or group of muscles flexing. You'll also be practicing mindful flexing and contracting of specific muscle groups in order to achieve a certain look or pose.

Weight lifting and bodybuilding promote muscle growth primarily through exercise focused on muscle shortening—concentric contraction with the goal to gain size (hypertrophy) and strength. Repetitive exercise of this sort, however, leads to tight muscles and restricted range of motion, which can take a toll on the joints and lead to injury. This impedes an athlete's ability to work to their full potential right up to a show or competition. Yoga poses work with movement through muscle lengthening—eccentric contraction—and promotes suppleness of the muscles, joint stability, and ease of movement. Yoga strengthens muscles by lengthening, keeping athletes moving freely through their available joint range. A restorative focus as part of a weight lifter or bodybuilder's regimen will help bring them to competition injury free with maximal gains.

Weight lifting or resistance training may include machines, free weights, bodyweight exercises, tubing, kettlebells, medicine balls, and so on. Regardless of the method practiced, it is prudent to ensure flexibility and fluidity of movement. Through these yoga poses, you can enhance your body awareness and mindful muscle recruitment, which is a vital component for a powerlifting or bodybuilding athlete. Likewise, practicing and understanding how muscles can be intentionally fired or activated during certain postures can enhance performance. These poses will also help you when you're striving for big or heavy lifts; you'll be more balanced and stable, resulting in power that is produced safely and effectively.

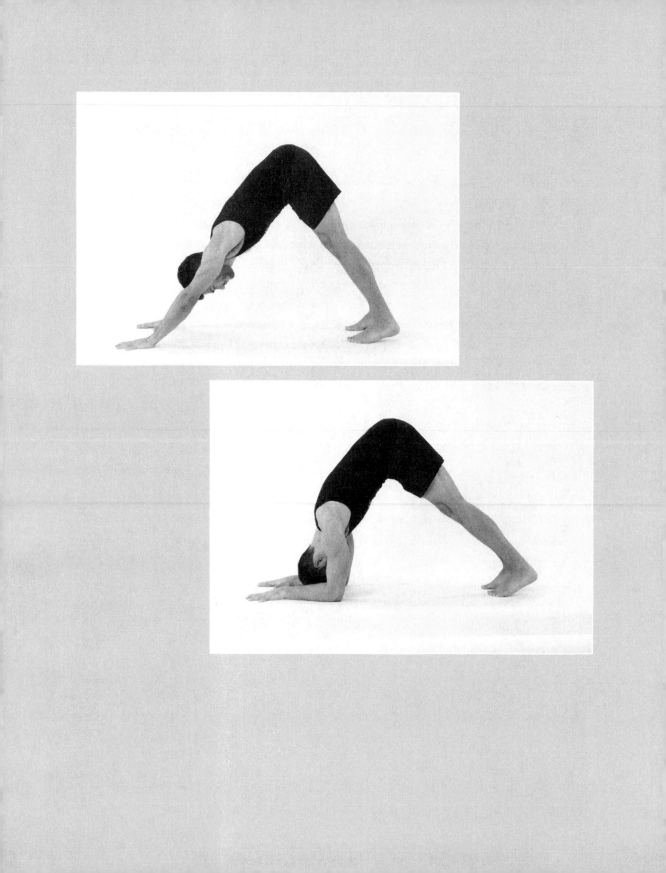

DOWNWARD FACING DOG/DOLPHIN

Benefit of Downward Facing Dog: This pose opens you across your chest and helps you breathe fully through your abdomen. It opens the front of your shoulders while building shoulder strength. It stretches the whole back of your body, including calves, hamstrings, glutes, and major back muscles. This pose releases tension in the body and, through the inversion effect, aids blood flow to your brain. It creates a sense of alertness to prepare you for what comes next. With regular practice this pose can also be very restful.

Benefit of Dolphin: Dolphin is sometimes preferred over Downward Facing Dog to ease tension in the wrists. It has the same benefits as Downward Facing Dog but with more intensity for the shoulders. You build more strength and increase your range of motion for weight lifting.

Getting into Downward Facing Dog: From Child's Pose, tuck your toes under and reach your arms ahead. Press into your toes and spread your fingers wide while you lift your hips to the sky. Make an inverted V shape with your body.

Getting into Dolphin: From Downward Facing Dog, lower onto your knees and bring your elbows directly under your shoulders. Press into your forearms and your toes and lift your hips high.

Holding the pose: Keep your head and neck relaxed and your shoulders away from your ears. Continue to lift your hips to the sky while you open your chest and shoulders down to your mat and breathe.

Modifications: If you have a hard time keeping your spine from rounding, bend your knees to keep your hips hinged and your spine long. Child's Pose is also an option for a rest at any time.

PLANK/FOREARM PLANK

Benefit of the pose: Plank challenges your whole torso, building strength and stability. It will strengthen your shoulders, chest, lower back, core, glutes, hamstrings, quads, and even muscles in your hands, wrists, feet, and ankles. Forearm Plank is nice for less intensity or to ease tension in your wrists.

Getting into the pose: From Downward Facing Dog, shift forward so that your shoulders are directly over your wrists into full Plank. From Dolphin, shift forward so that your shoulders are directly over your elbows into Forearm Plank. Lower your hips so that you form one long line from your ankles to your shoulders.

Holding the pose: Press through your heels and engage your quads and inner thighs. Lift your core center and stabilize your shoulders. Reach through the crown of your head and spread the work through your entire body.

Modifications: To ease tension and reduce intensity, move to a kneeling position for both Plank options.

Option to flow: From Downward Facing Dog, inhale and shift forward into Plank and, as you exhale, shift back to Downward Facing Dog. From Dolphin, inhale and shift forward to Forearm Plank and exhale back to Dolphin.

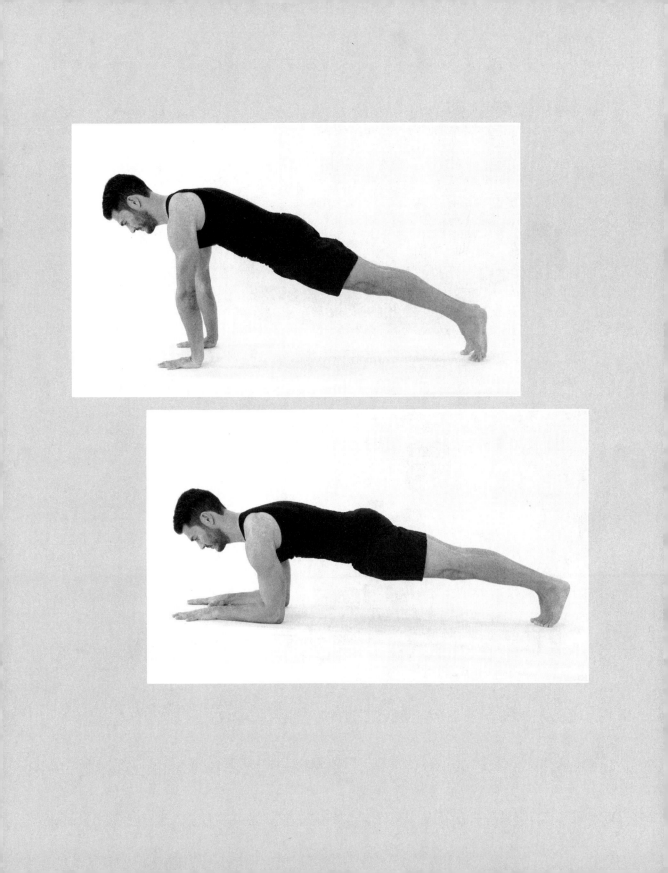

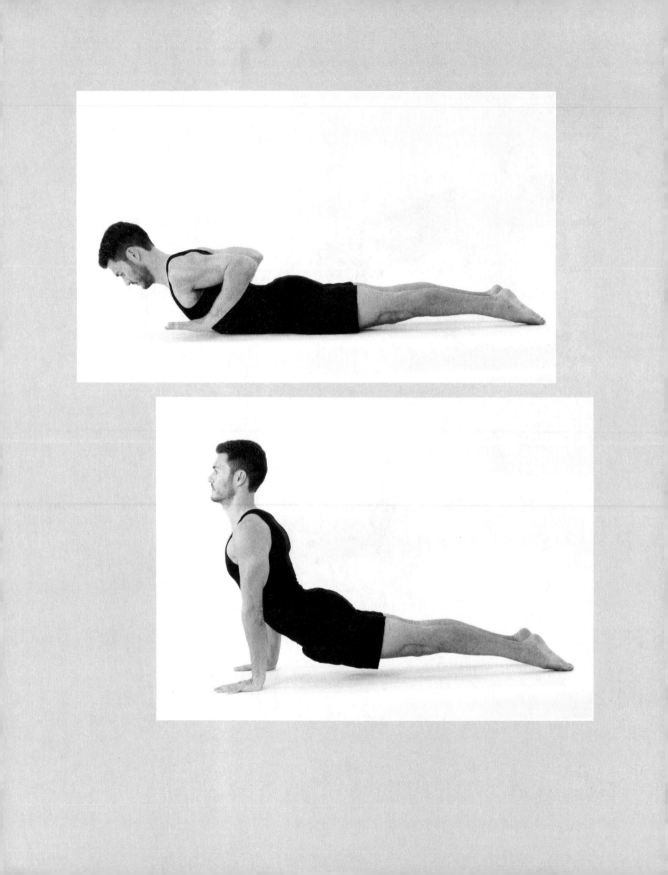

COBRA/UPWARD FACING DOG

Benefit of the pose: Both of these poses strengthen your upper back when lifting. They also strengthen your core center and lower back extensors while stretching your chest and shoulders. Cobra prepares you for more intense back work, while Upward Facing Dog is the more intense option, focusing on your shoulders.

Getting into Cobra: From Plank or Kneeling Plank, bring your body to the floor and keep your hands under your shoulders. Engage your inner thighs and pelvic floor and draw your belly button to your spine. Pull your shoulder blades toward your spine and reach through the crown of your head while you lift your chest and shoulders off the mat.

Getting into Upward Facing Dog: From Crocodile/Plank, flip your feet so that the tops of your feet are pressing into the mat. Reach through the crown of your head and pull your heart forward. Lower your pelvis but keep your legs off the mat. Lengthen your arms and reach your shoulders back and down. Engage your pelvic floor and core to protect your lower back.

Holding the pose: Continue to lengthen from head to toe while you lift your navel toward your spine and draw your shoulders back and down. In Cobra, instead of pushing up with your hands, let your back muscles lift you up. In Upward Facing Dog, press away from your mat to support your weight and continue to pull your heart forward.

Modifications: If Upward Facing Dog is too much, choose Cobra. Feel free to rest back in Child's Pose if this brings on fatigue.

MONKEY

Benefit of the pose: This pose strengthens the entire back, rear shoulder muscles, core center, glutes, and hamstrings. This movement is necessary for safe and effective deadlifts in the weight room. It develops proper form and perhaps an awareness of faulty movement patterns.

Getting into the pose: From forward fold, place your hands on your shins. With a micro bend in your knees, reach your heart forward.

Holding the pose: Continue to reach through the crown of your head and your tailbone to lengthen your spine. Reach your shoulders back and down and imagine a flattened back.

Modifications: Bend your knees more to ease tension through your hamstrings and lower back. For more release, place your hands on your thighs or on a block in front of you for more support while you build strength.

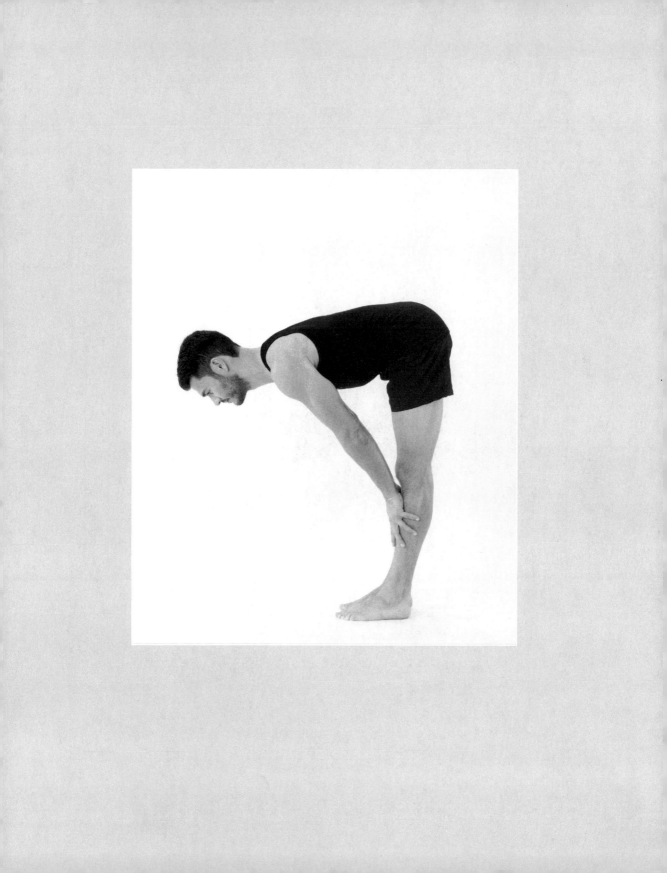

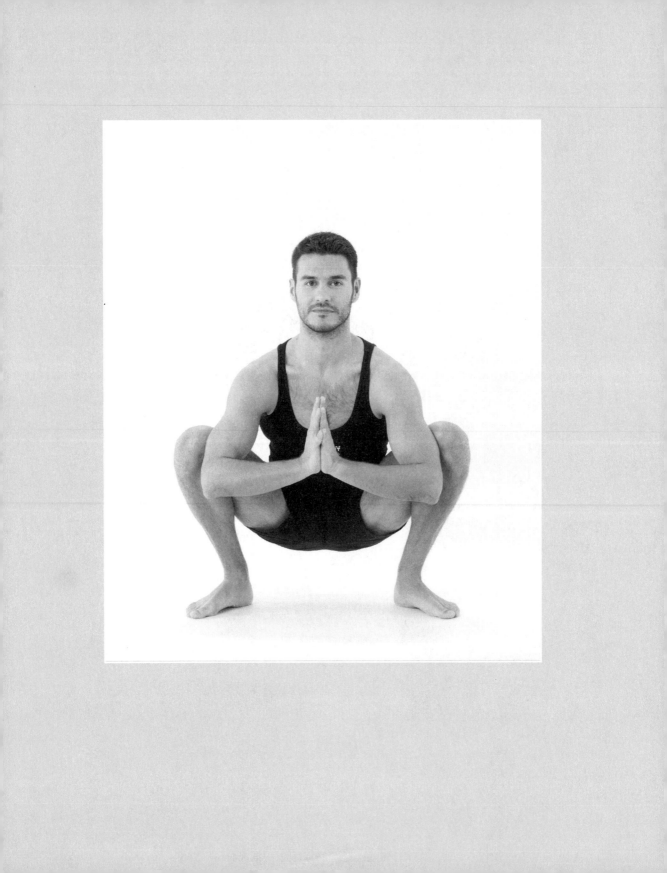

GARLAND

Benefit of the pose: Essentially a deep squat, Garland strengthens your hips, thighs, and upper back muscles. It is very functional for getting up and down from the floor and increases your range of motion in your hips while releasing tension.

Getting into the pose: From Monkey, release to a forward fold and shuffle your feet outward to a comfortable position. Place your hands or elbows on your thighs and lower your hips toward the floor, keeping a neutral spine. Adjust your foot position as necessary to keep your whole foot on the floor. As you lower your hips below the knees, keep your upper body raised, heart open.

Holding the pose: Work your upper back to stay lifted in your spine. Shift your weight from foot to foot and adjust their position so that your feet, ankles, and calves are comfortable. Stay extended in the upper spine.

Modifications: If you tend to round your back, keep your pelvis a little higher (level with your knees) and your hands on your thighs. Gradually work to lower your pelvis a little more. Roll or fold a mat to form a wedge and place it under your heels so that your feet and calves may relax.

BOW

Benefit of the pose: Bow opens up the whole front side of the body—quads, hip flexors, abdominals, chest, and shoulders—while strengthening the entire back side of the body, including your hamstrings, glutes, back extensors, and upper back. Performed with intense levels of exertion, it helps the body to release tension and pent-up energy. This pose is great for offsetting excessive amounts of forward flexion (rounding of the spine and shoulders).

Getting into the pose: Lie on your belly and open your shoulders to reach behind to your ankles. Flex your feet and draw your thighs inward. Press your ankles into your hands and hold your ankles firmly. Engage your core center and lift away from the body.

Holding the pose: Keep a strong core center and continue to lift through the crown of your head and press your ankles into your hands.

Modifications: If you have difficulty getting both hands to your ankles, use Half Bow, which is performed one side at a time. Place one arm in front of you bent at the elbow. Use your hand and forearm across your mat for support and reach your other hand to the ankle on the same side. Another option is to place a strap around your ankle and hold on to the strap.

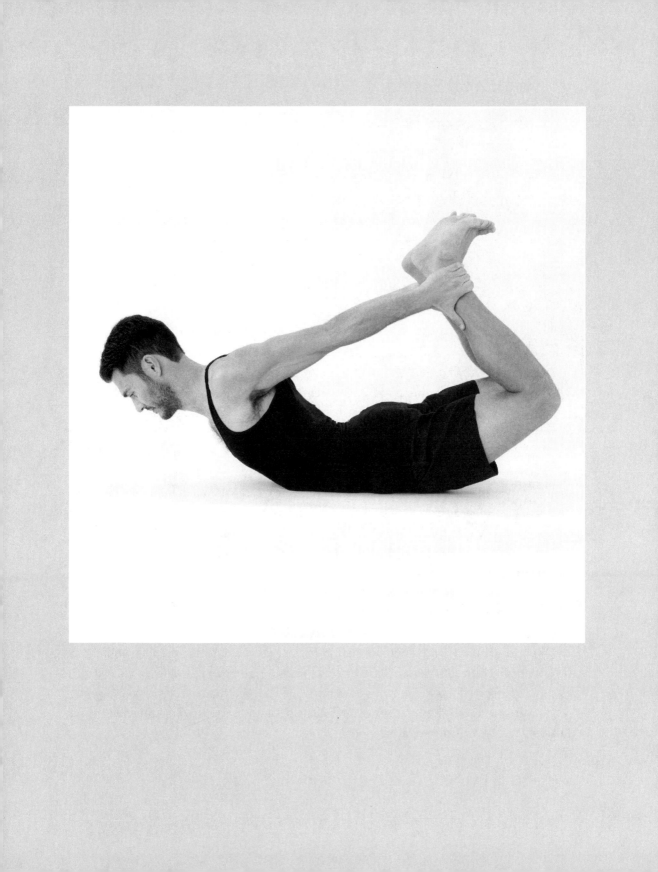

Kickboxing/Boxing

Kickboxing and boxing are similar in obvious ways. The difference is that kickboxing allows hands *and* feet (and sometimes knees) as a defense. In both, however, hips are the prime power and mobility center, generating a lot of force from the legs, up through the torso, and out the arms. A strong boxer will leverage the whole body to produce a power hit that registers from foot to fingertip. That, combined with a keen awareness to dodge hits, means that you can become tense for long periods of time unless mindfully relaxing when the opportunity arises.

Whether you are in the ring, contact boxing, or regularly attend a kickboxing or shadowboxing class, your repetitive arm movements, blocks, punches, and bouncing from side to side can leave you with upper cross tightness. Poses aimed to open the chest and shoulders can help balance, strength, and flexibility along with reducing tightness. Furthermore, lower leg stretches and any inversions with a focus on breath can help alleviate compression and tightness in your hips and lower back caused by the quick footwork known as "the boxer bounce."

Kickboxers will also benefit from poses including Camel and Bow as they open the front of the body and lengthen the hip flexors, quadriceps, abdominals, and chest. These will help with your forward kick motion and load-bearing single leg balancing.

When practicing a punch for power, you are coached to forcefully exhale to generate greater power. My breath exercises will help you to control your breath and connect with this type of forceful exhalation.

These sports require full engagement of the mind; they are as much mental games as physical endeavors. You have to predict the next punch from your opponent and plan your next move while at the same time getting out of your head in order to bring full concentration to these aspects. Injuries are often a result of impact from hits, and you have to be alert, responsive, and guarded to protect yourself and prepare for your counterattack. This is a lot of mental stimulation, so it is worthwhile to work with grounding, calming energy as well. Once you learn how to connect with your mind through yoga practice, you will be able to channel your focus in the ring.

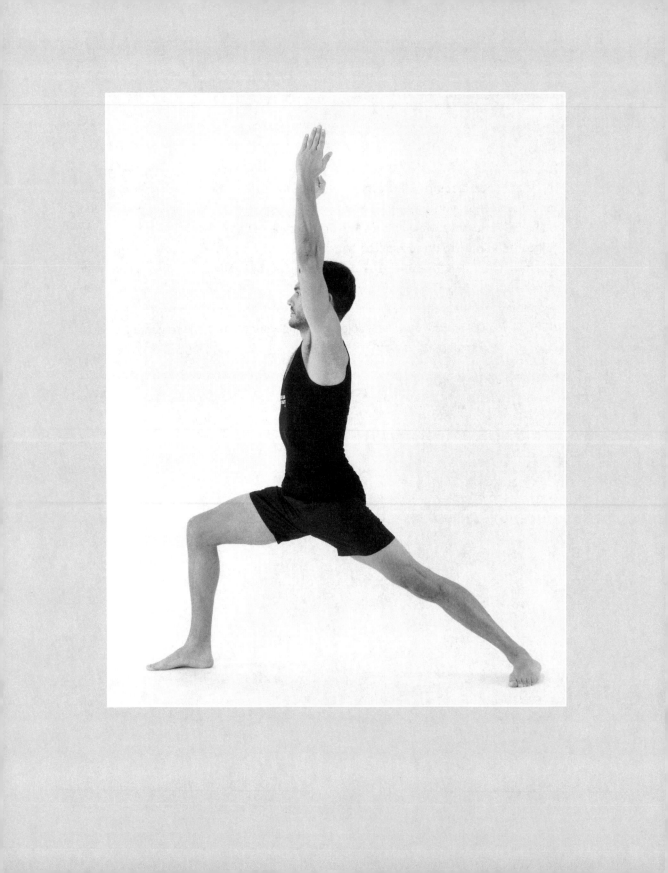

WARRIOR I / WARRIOR LUNGE

Benefit of the pose: This pose opens up the front of your hips on one side while strengthening your hip and thigh muscles on the other. Upper back muscles are also strengthened by staying lifted through the heart. Warrior poses help to keep our hips mobile and strong.

Getting into the pose: From a standing position, step back with one foot and extend your arms above with your shoulders back and down. For Warrior I, lower your back heel to the floor, keeping your pelvis facing forward. For Warrior Lunge, keep your back heel lifted.

Holding the pose: In Warrior I, straighten your back leg and keep all four corners of your back foot on your mat. Feel the work in your pelvis. In Warrior Lunge, keep your front knee over your ankle and press through your back heel to open your hip.

Modifications: If you feel tension in your lower back in Warrior I, lift your heel into Warrior Lunge or step wider side to side to make room to move your pelvis. For less sensation in Warrior Lunge, take your back knee to the floor and place your hands on your front thigh.

WARRIOR II

Benefit of the pose: Warrior II stretches inner thighs and calves while strengthening the quads, glutes, hamstrings, upper back, and shoulders. It increases your ability to deal with stress and improves your focus.

Getting into the pose: From Warrior I/Warrior Lunge, keep your front knee over the ankle. Inhale and lift your body slightly upward and rotate your torso open to the long edge of your mat. Look over your front fingers as you lower your body.

Holding the pose: Reach forward and back with your arms and keep your pelvis directly beneath your ribs. Continue to notice your knee and make sure it stays over the front ankle. Engage your core center and lift through the top of your head to stay long through your torso. Relax your shoulders back and down.

Modifications: For less intensity, shorten your stance and be up a little higher. To relieve tension in the neck and shoulders bring your hands to your heart.

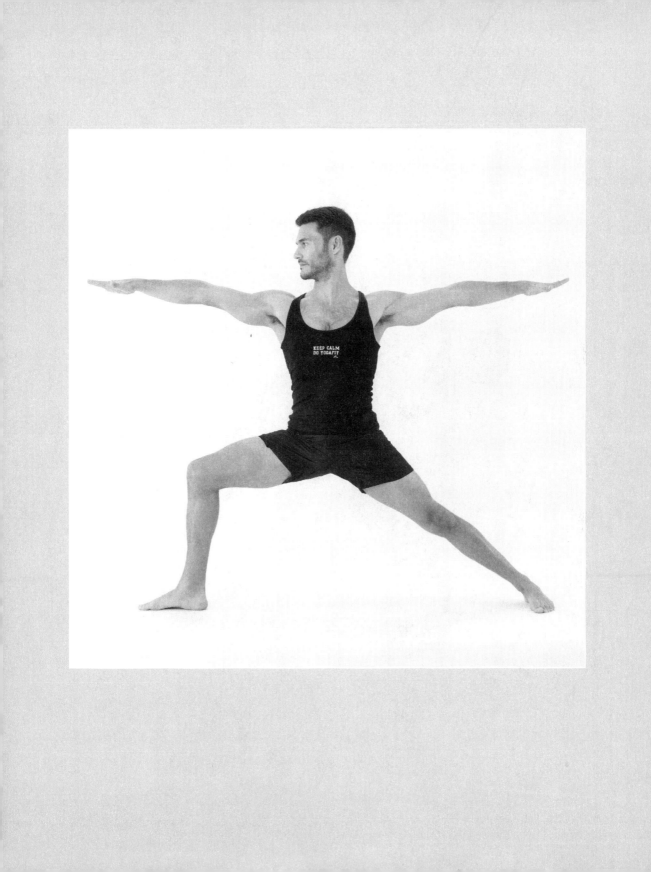

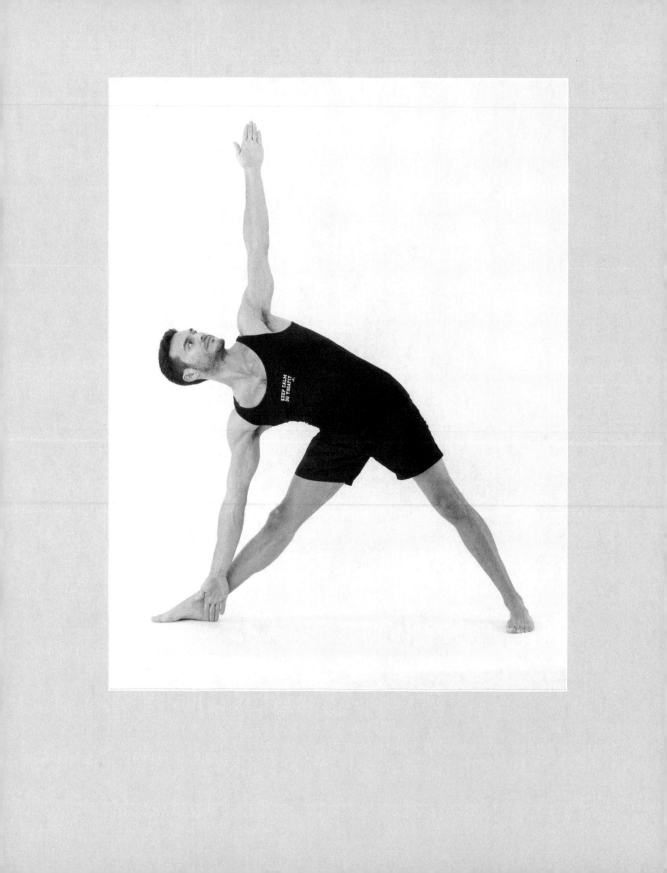

TRIANGLE

Benefit of the pose: Triangle works with Warrior poses to stretch and strengthen your groin. It targets hamstrings and inner thighs for a great stretch and strengthens your quads, obliques, hip flexors, and rear shoulders.

Getting into the pose: From Warrior II, reach forward with your front arm while you lengthen your front leg with a micro bend in your front knee. Keep your side body long; your spine does not flex down. Reach your arms to the earth and sky.

Holding the pose: Engage your glutes to bring your hips in line with your legs. Rotate your torso upward and continue to reach to the earth and sky and reach through the crown of your head.

Modifications: For less sensation, lower your top hand to your hip. If you are rounding to the floor, place a block under your hand for support. Do this pose against a wall to feel where your hips, shoulders, and head should align.

DOWNWARD FACING DOG

Benefit of the pose: This pose opens you across your chest and helps you breathe fully through your abdomen. It opens the front of your shoulders while building shoulder strength. It stretches the whole back of your body, including calves, hamstrings, glutes, and major back muscles. This pose releases tension in the body and, through the inversion effect, aids blood flow to your brain. It creates a sense of alertness to prepare you for what comes next. With regular practice this pose can also be very restful.

Getting into the pose: From Child's Pose, tuck your toes under and reach your arms ahead. Press into your toes and spread your fingers wide while you lift your hips to the sky. Make an inverted V shape with your body.

Holding the pose: Inhale to reach your tailbone up and lengthen your spine. Exhale to bring your chest and belly toward your thighs.

Modifications: If you have a hard time keeping your spine from rounding, bend your knees to keep your hips hinged and your spine long. To relieve tension in your wrists, come down onto the forearms with your elbows shoulder-width apart. Child's Pose is also an option for a rest at any time.

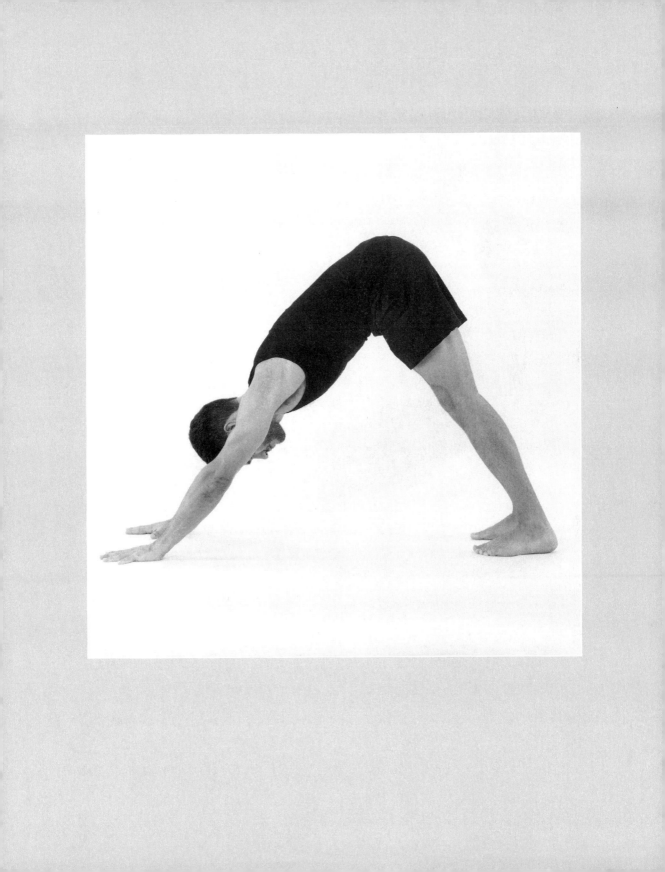

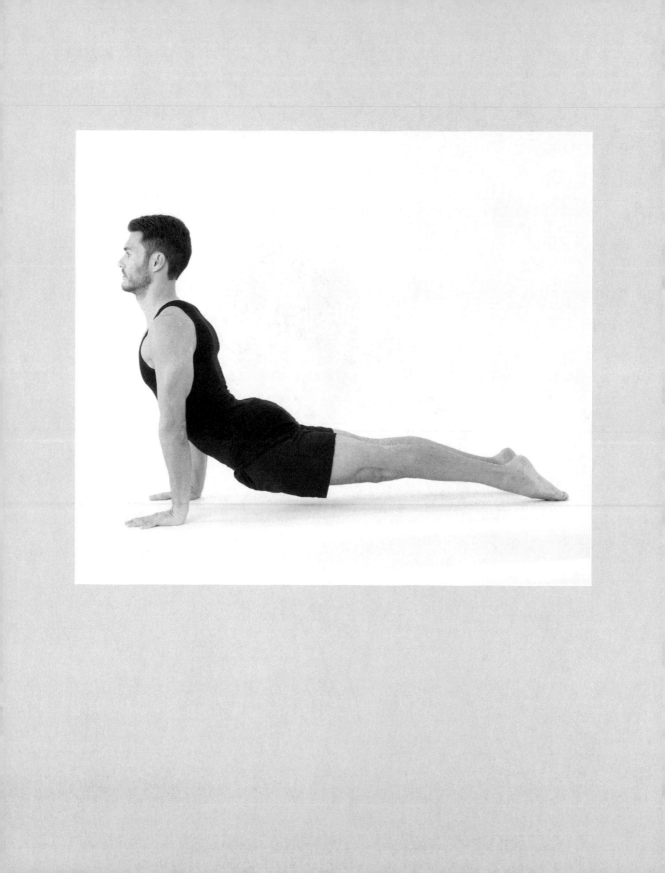

UPWARD FACING DOG or HALF SERIES

Benefit of the pose: Upward Facing Dog strengthens the entire back, lower chest muscles, triceps, and your core center. It also stretches your upper chest and shoulders. Upward Facing Dog is a great pose on its own for strength or in a flow, as in Half Series, seen on page 40, which will help power and increase intensity in your chest and shoulders.

Getting into Upward Facing Dog: From Downward Facing Dog, shift forward into Plank and flip your feet so that the tops of your feet are pressing into the mat. Reach through the crown of your head and pull your heart forward. Lower your pelvis but keep your legs off of the mat. Lengthen your arms and reach your shoulders back and down. Engage your pelvic floor and core to protect your lower back.

Holding the pose: Continue to lengthen from head to toe while you lift your navel toward your spine and draw your shoulders back and down. Press away from your mat to support your weight and continue to pull your heart forward.

Modifications: For less intensity, choose Cobra Pose or the Kneeling Half Series, page 40. Feel free to rest back in Child's Pose in the case of fatigue.

CAMEL

Benefit of the pose: This pose opens up the entire front of your body. It stretches quads, hip flexors, chest, and shoulders while strengthening hamstrings, glutes, and the upper and lower back. It helps to lift your mood and reduce stress.

Getting into the pose: From a kneeling position, lift your hips directly over your knees. Open your chest and shoulders and place your fists or palms on the back side of your pelvis. Press your pelvis forward by firming your glutes. Extend open through your heart and the crown of your head.

Holding the pose: Continue to lift your heart up and create space in your lower back. Extend farther where you can and reach for your heels. When reaching for your heels, do not twist or lower your hips.

Modifications: For less sensation, bring your palms back to your pelvis. You may also come to the floor and use Cobra or Locust. In Locust, try reaching your hands behind you and interlacing your fingers.

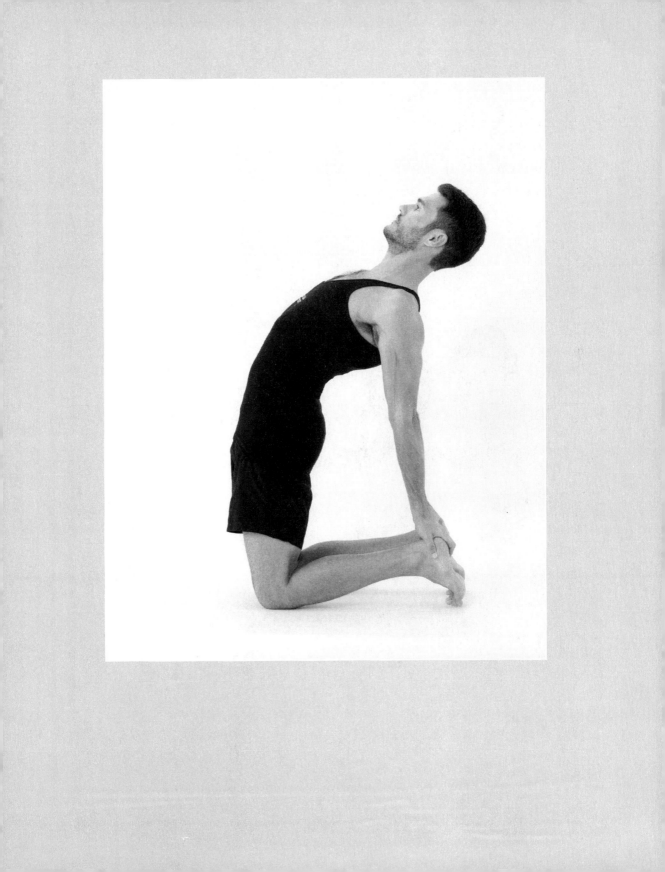

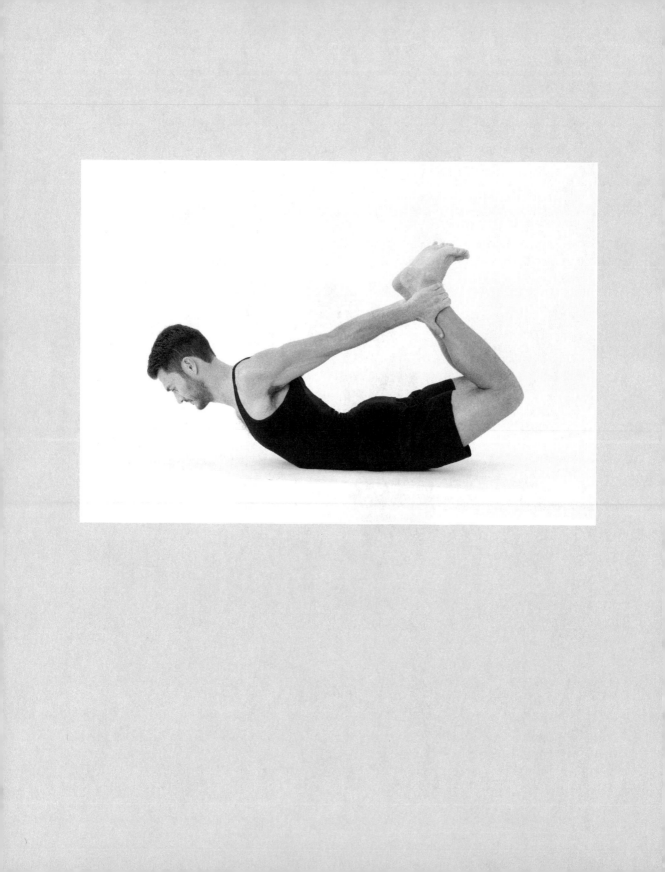

BOW

Benefit of the pose: Bow opens up the whole front side of the body—quads, hip flexors, abdominals, chest, and shoulders—while strengthening the entire back side of the body, including your hamstrings, glutes, back extensors, and upper back. Performed with intense levels of exertion, it helps the body to release tension and pent-up energy. This pose is great for offsetting excessive amounts of forward flexion (rounding of the spine and shoulders).

Getting into the pose: Lie on your belly and open your shoulders to reach behind to your ankles. Flex your feet and draw your thighs inward. Press your ankles into your hands and hold firmly while you lift up and away from your body.

Holding the pose: Inhale and lengthen your spine from your tailbone to the crown of your head. Exhale and focus on strength throughout the back, inner thighs, and core center.

Modifications: If you have difficulty getting both hands to your ankles, use Half Bow, which is performed one side at a time. Place one arm in front of you bent at the elbow. Use your hand and forearm across your mat for support and reach your other hand to the ankle on the same side. Another option is to place a strap around your ankle and hold on to the strap.

CHILD'S POSE

Benefit of the pose: Child's Pose is often used to offset the intensity of intense back extensions, a counter pose. Child's Pose is grounding, relaxing, and soothing to the body physically and energetically. When sports activity demands high levels of intensity, alertness, action, and reaction, levels of cortisol (a stress hormone) rise. Child's Pose is very restorative.

Getting into the pose: From your belly, press back to bring your hips toward your heels. From a kneeling position, reach your hands out in front on the floor and lower your body to your thighs.

Holding the pose: Your arms can stay over your head or you can put them along your sides. Use your breath and gravity to relax and let go. With your arms overhead, you can easily make transitions into other poses.

Modifications: Widen your knees to clear space for your belly. If your hips or knees are uncomfortable, place some padding under or behind your knees. You may also leave your hips up higher to relieve tension.

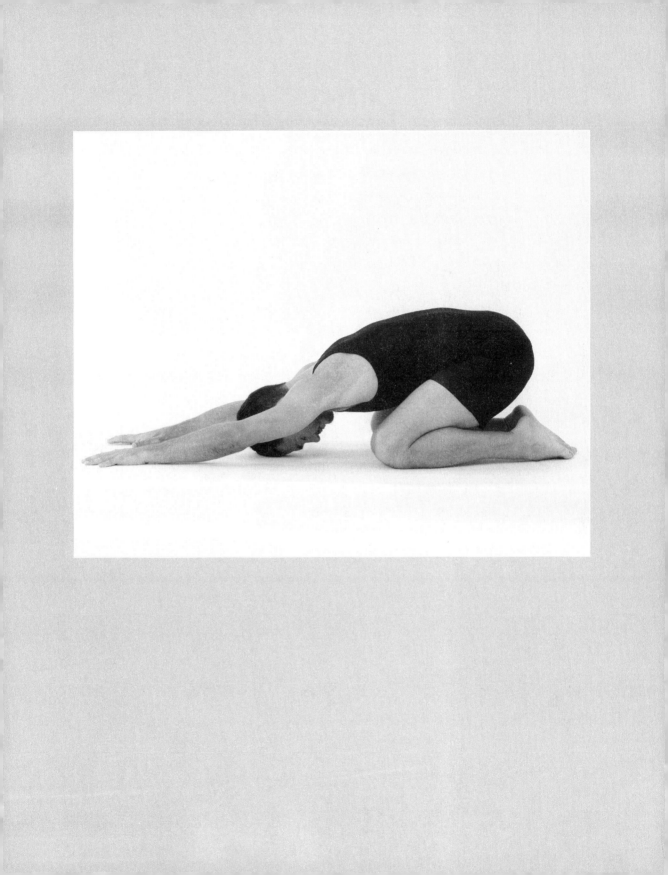

CrossFit

A hugely popular and community-based sport, CrossFit focuses on different body parts throughout the week with daily Workout of the Day (WOD) routines. Combined, these daily routines develop and work the entire body. CrossFit is based on some of the same exercises you see with weight lifters and power lifters—Olympic lifting, snatches, and so on—and depending on your goal, you will either train for time (how quickly you can perform the WODs) or train for a fit body.

If training for time, you need to be careful because lifting heavy weight at intense speed can result in careless and jerky movements. Doing this repetitively over time without slowing down will increase the chance of injury. This yoga sequence is intended to support the CrossFit moves and avoid tightness and is primarily designed to help you recover and prepare your body for the next WOD.

In addition to the core exercises in your CrossFit workouts, my controlled Plank or

Side Plank can help with strengthening the core, powering up your pull-ups, rope climbs, and medicine ball slams. Yoga's focus on breath and mental agility will also up your CrossFit performance, given the high-intensity challenges you'll face and the mental game of digging deep to reach your personal best for reps or time. The intensity of CrossFit and the calm, slow nature of yoga are the perfect yin/yang pairing!

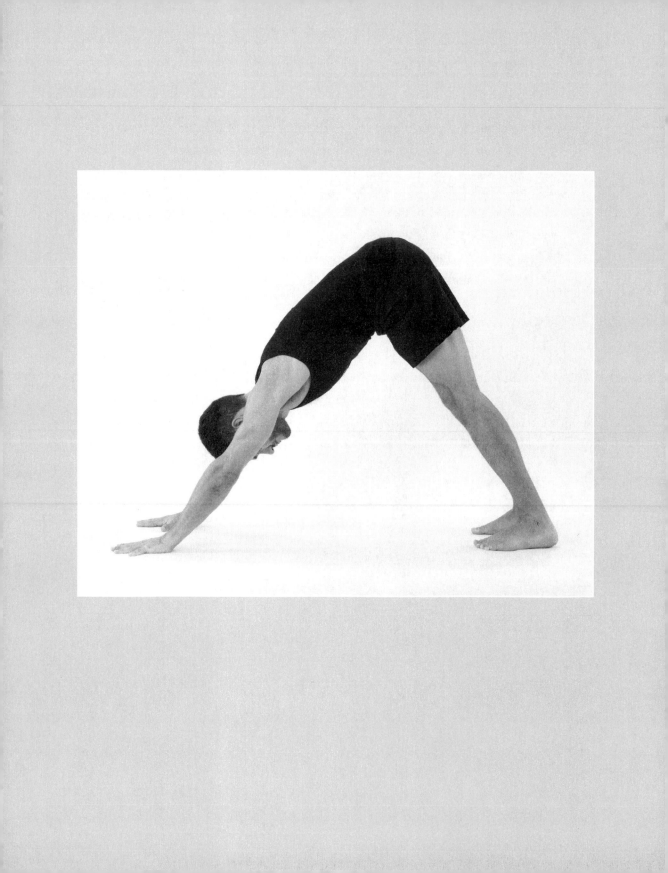

DOWNWARD FACING DOG

Benefit of the pose: This pose opens you across your chest and helps you breathe fully through your abdomen. It opens the front of your shoulders while building shoulder strength. It stretches the whole back of your body, including calves, hamstrings, glutes, and major back muscles. This pose releases tension in the body and, through the inversion effect, aids blood flow to your brain. It creates a sense of alertness to prepare you for what comes next. With regular practice this pose can also be very restful.

Getting into the pose: From Child's Pose, tuck your toes under and reach your arms ahead. Press into your toes and spread your fingers wide while you lift your hips to the sky. Make an inverted V shape with your body.

Holding the pose: Inhale to reach your tailbone up and lengthen your spine. Exhale to bring your chest and belly toward your thighs.

Modifications: If you have a hard time keeping your spine from rounding, bend your knees to keep your hips hinged and your spine long. To relieve tension in your wrists, come down onto the forearms with your elbows shoulder-width apart. Child's Pose is also an option for a rest at any time.

UPWARD FACING DOG or HALF SERIES

Benefit of the pose: Upward Facing Dog strengthens the entire back, lower chest muscles, triceps, and your core center. It also stretches your upper chest and shoulders. Upward Facing Dog is great to use as a flow, as in Half Series, page 40, a more intense option with more work in your shoulders.

Getting into Upward Facing Dog: From Downward Facing Dog, shift forward into Plank and flip your feet so that the tops of your feet are pressing into the mat. Reach through the crown of your head and pull your heart forward. Lower your pelvis but keep your legs off of the mat. Lengthen your arms and reach your shoulders back and down. Engage your pelvic floor and core to protect your lower back.

Holding the pose: Continue to lengthen from head to toe while you lift your navel toward your spine and draw your shoulders back and down. Press away from your mat to support your weight and continue to pull your heart forward.

Modifications: For less intensity, choose Cobra Pose or the Kneeling Half Series, page 42. Feel free to rest back in Child's Pose in case of fatigue.

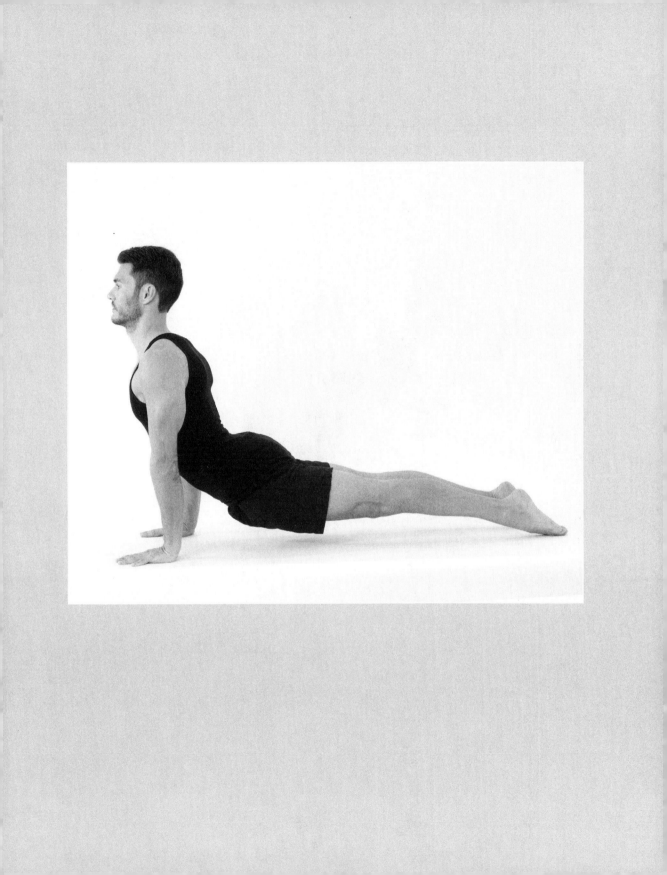

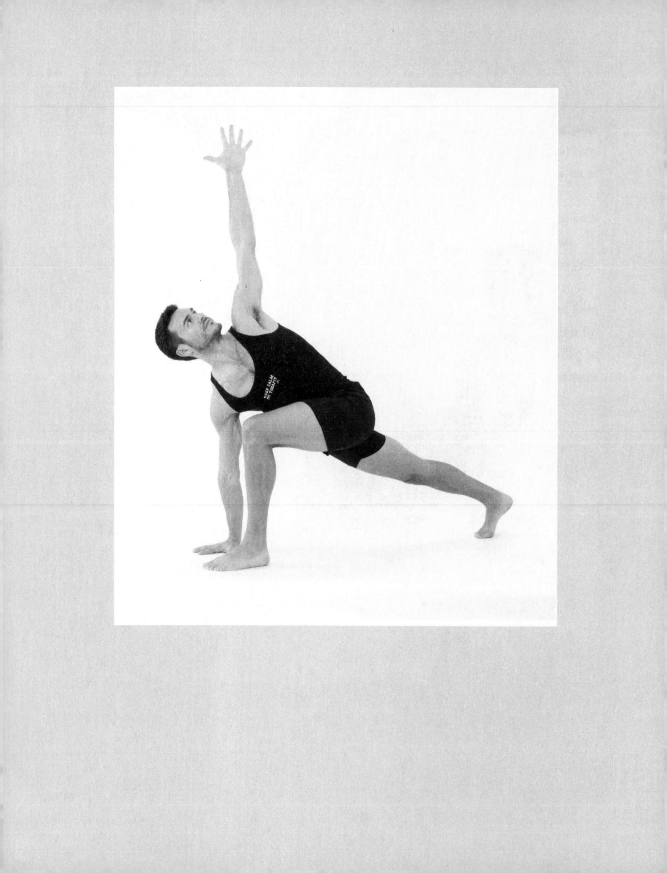

TWISTING LUNGE

Benefit of the pose: Like Warrior Lunge, this pose opens the front of your hips and strengthens your knees, quads, and upper back. The twist strengthens your hip adductors and obliques on one side while stretching them on the opposite side. The twist invigorates your muscles through your whole torso, stimulating conductivity of your sensory nerves and massaging your internal organs.

Getting into the pose: From a Warrior Lunge, lengthen through the crown of your head and keep your spine long. Engage your core center and twist first with your navel, then your chest, then your shoulders toward your front leg.

Holding the pose: Keep one hand on the floor for support and lift the other to the sky. For more sensation, bring your lower arm across your front thigh and bring both hands to your heart. Continue to lengthen your spine, rotate further, and press into your back heel to deepen the posture.

Modifications: You can perform this posture with your back knee down on the mat—with extra padding under your knee for more comfort. You may also place your floor hand on a block for support, which may help to extend your spine.

CAMEL

Benefit of the pose: This pose opens up the entire front of your body. It stretches quads, hip flexors, chest, and shoulders while strengthening hamstrings, glutes, and the upper and lower back. It helps to lift your mood and reduce stress.

Getting into the pose: From a kneeling position, lift your hips directly over your knees. Open your chest and shoulders and place your fists or palms on the back side of your pelvis. Press your pelvis forward by firming your glutes. Extend open through your heart and the crown of your head.

Holding the pose: Continue to lift your heart up and create space in your lower back. Extend farther where you can and reach for your heels. When reaching for your heels, do not twist or lower your hips.

Modifications: For less sensation, bring your palms back to your pelvis. You may also come to the floor and use Cobra or Locust. In Locust, try reaching your hands behind you and interlacing your fingers.

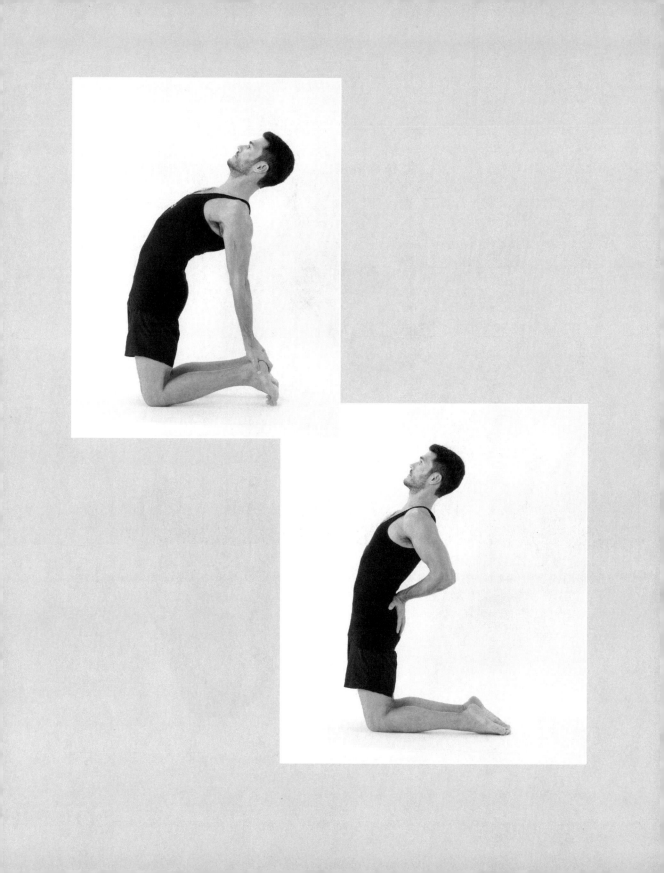

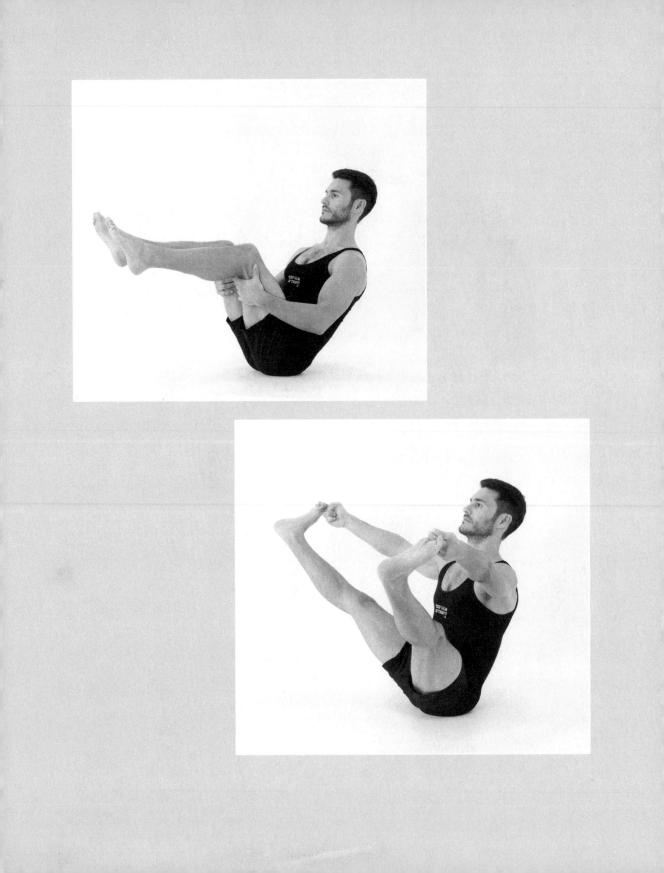

BOAT/WIDE BOAT

Benefit of the pose: This pose strengthens your abdominals, upper back, hip flexors, and quads. Your core center stabilizes you while you strengthen your upper back to stay lifted.

Getting into the pose: From a seated position, bend your knees and place your feet flat on the floor. Sit tall with your spine long and place your hands just behind your knees. Lean back and sit just behind your sitting bones. Maintain a long spine and lift one leg at a time off your mat.

Holding the pose: Focus on your core center and keep your spine long. When you are ready, reach your arms away from your legs. Reach your arms forward or up for more sensation. For Wide Boat, lengthen your legs up and out to the side, even taking hold of your toes for hand-to-toe hold.

Modifications: Move one foot at a time off of your mat or keep both feet on your mat for support. To ease tension or prevent rounding in the lower back, continue to hold behind the knees.

INCLINE PLANK/TABLE TOP

Benefit of the pose: Both of these poses strengthen your glutes, hamstrings, inner thighs, rear shoulders, triceps, and your core center. They also stretch the front of your shoulders, chest, and hip flexors.

Getting into Incline Plank: From a seated position, place your hands directly under your shoulders, fingers pointing toward your feet. Pull your shoulder blades back and open your chest. Reach your legs long on your mat with your feet hip distance apart. Press into your heels and lift your hips to the sky. Create a long line between your feet and the crown of your head.

Getting into Table Top: Bend your knees and place your feet flat on your mat. Press your feet into your mat and lift your hips to the sky.

Holding the pose: In Incline Plank, gently roll your feet inward to prevent your legs from rolling out. In Table Top, you're engaging your inner thighs to align your knees over your ankles. Keep your gaze up without dropping your head back.

Modifications: If you want to relieve tension in your hips and lower back, choose Table Top. If you want to relieve tension in your shoulders, choose Incline Plank. To relieve tension in your hips and shoulders, keep your hips down and stay lifted in your chest and shoulders, or you can lower yourself to your mat and lift just the hips into Bridge, see page 191.

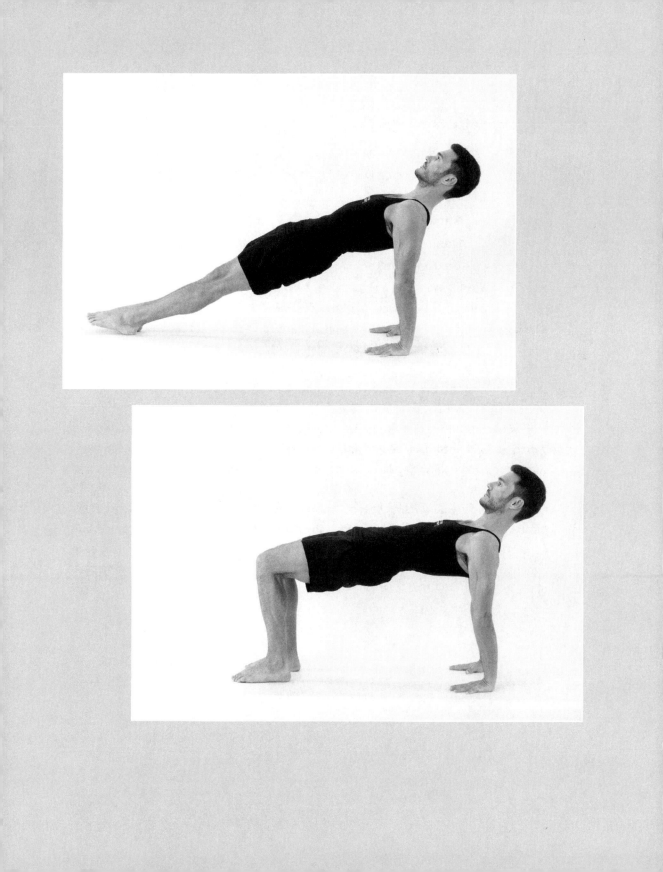

Cycling

Bicycling is low-impact, gentle on the joints. But cyclists are predominantly in a bent-forward (or forward flex) position and are quad-dominant, which leads to tight hip flexors. A series of poses that trigger hip opening, hip flexor, and hamstring stretches will help balance this out. The Downward Facing Dog and Upward Facing Dog combinations will provide essential movement and extension to open up the chest and shoulders at the same time.

If you choose to take on mountain biking and trails that pose uneven ground and speed, you will need balance and agility to handle the required unpredictable maneuvers. Poses that help with balance and core control will give you needed strength and stability on the bike.

To achieve greater cycling speed, the entire pedal stroke must be productive. This means that the push on the front end of the pedal stroke is complemented by the pull on the back side. But as you lift your heel to transfer into another push, you can have tight hamstrings. Downward Facing Dog will feel good—it will help lengthen the back of your legs.

DOWNWARD FACING DOG

Benefit of the pose: This pose opens you across your chest and helps you breathe fully through your abdomen. It opens the front of your shoulders while building shoulder strength. It stretches the whole back of your body, including calves, hamstrings, glutes, and major back muscles. This pose releases tension in the body and, through the inversion effect, aids blood flow to your brain. It creates a sense of alertness to prepare you for what comes next. With regular practice this pose can also be very restful.

Getting into the pose: From Child's Pose, tuck your toes under and reach your arms ahead. Press into your toes and spread your fingers wide while you lift your hips to the sky. Make an inverted V shape with your body.

Holding the pose: Inhale to reach your tailbone up and lengthen your spine. Exhale to bring your chest and belly toward your thighs.

Modifications: If you have a hard time keeping your spine from rounding, bend your knees to keep your hips hinged and your spine long. To relieve tension in your wrists, come down onto the forearms with your elbows shoulder-width apart. Child's Pose is also an option for a rest at any time.

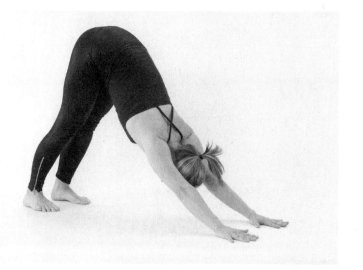

UPWARD FACING DOG or HALF SERIES

Benefit of the pose: Upward Facing Dog strengthens the entire back, lower chest muscles, triceps, and your core center. It also stretches your upper chest and shoulders. Upward Facing Dog is great to use as a flow as in Half Series, page 40, a more intense option with more work in your shoulders.

Getting into Upward Facing Dog: From Downward Facing Dog, shift forward into Plank and flip your feet so that the tops of your feet are pressing into the mat. Reach through the crown of your head and pull your heart forward. Lower your pelvis but keep your legs off of the mat. Lengthen your arms and reach your shoulders back and down. Engage your pelvic floor and core to protect your lower back.

Holding the pose: Continue to lengthen from head to toe while you lift your navel toward your spine and draw your shoulders back and down. Press away from your mat to support your weight and continue to pull your heart forward.

Modifications: For less intensity, choose Cobra Pose or the Kneeling Half Series, page 42. Feel free to rest back in Child's Pose in the case of fatigue.

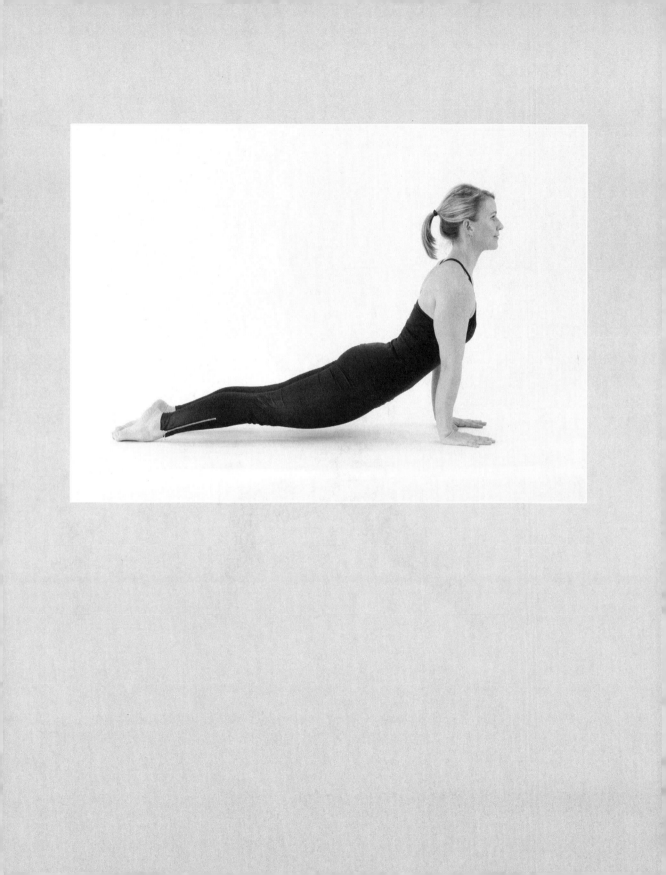

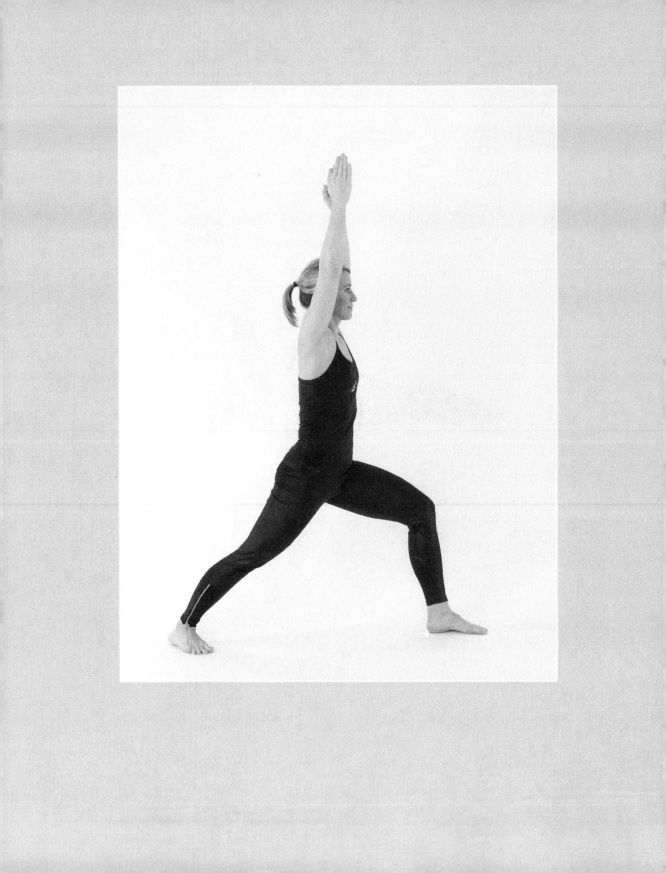

WARRIOR I

Benefit of the pose: This pose opens up the front of your hips on one side while strengthening your hip and thigh muscles on the other. Upper back muscles are also strengthened by staying lifted through the heart. Warrior poses help to keep our hips mobile and strong.

Getting into the pose: From a standing position, step back with one foot and extend your arms above with your shoulders back and down. Lower your back heel to the floor, keeping your pelvis facing forward.

Holding the pose: Straighten your leg and keep all four corners of your back foot on your mat. Feel the work in the pelvis.

Modifications: If you feel tension in your lower back, lift your heel as in Warrior Lunge or step wider side to side to make room to move your pelvis.

WARRIOR II

Benefit of the pose: Warrior II stretches inner thighs and calves while strengthening the quads, glutes, hamstrings, upper back, and shoulders. It increases your ability to deal with stress and improves your focus.

Getting into the pose: From Warrior I, keep your front knee over the ankle. Inhale and lift your body slightly upward and rotate your torso open to the long edge of your mat. Look over your front fingers as you lower your body.

Holding the pose: Reach forward and back with your arms and keep your pelvis directly beneath your ribs. Continue to notice your knee and make sure it stays over the front ankle. Engage your core center and lift through the top of your head to stay long through your torso. Relax your shoulders back and down.

Modifications: For less intensity, shorten your stance and be up a little higher. To relieve tension in the neck and shoulders, bring your hands to your heart.

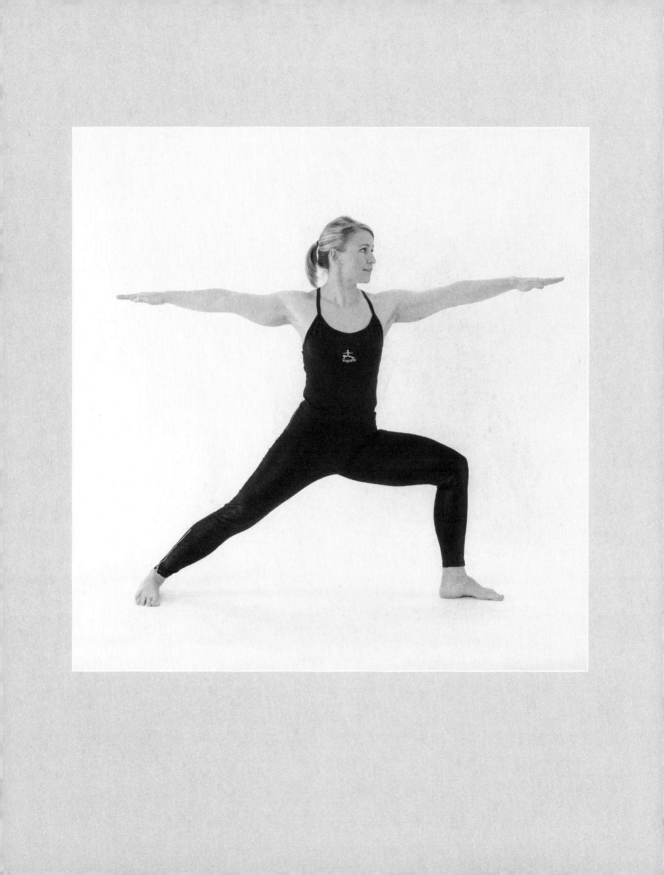

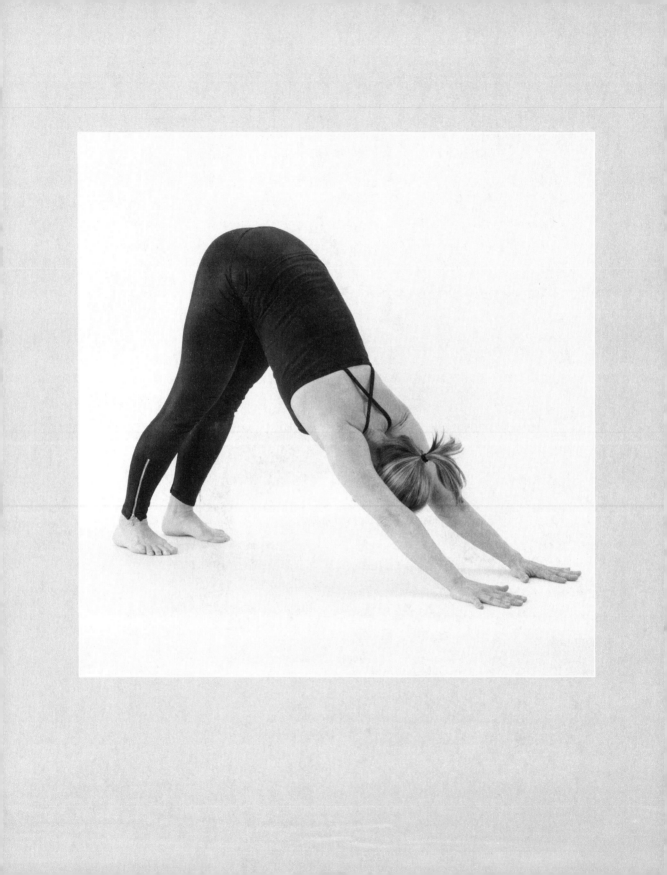

DOWNWARD FACING DOG

Benefit of the pose: This pose opens you across your chest and helps you breathe fully through your abdomen. It opens the front of your shoulders while building shoulder strength. It stretches the whole back of your body, including calves, hamstrings, glutes, and major back muscles. This pose releases tension in the body and, through the inversion effect, aids blood flow to your brain. It creates a sense of alertness to prepare you for what comes next. With regular practice this pose can be very restful.

Getting into the pose: From Warrior II, windmill your hands to the floor and step back to Downward Facing Dog. Press into your toes and spread your fingers wide while you lift your hips to the sky. Make an inverted V shape with your body.

Holding the pose: Inhale to reach your tailbone up and lengthen your spine. Exhale to bring your chest and belly toward your thighs.

Modifications: If you have a hard time keeping your spine from rounding, bend your knees to keep your hips hinged and your spine long. To relieve tension in your wrists, come down onto the forearms with your elbows shoulder-width apart. Child's Pose is also an option for a rest at any time.

LOCUST

Benefit of the pose: This pose strengthens the entire back of the body, including your hamstrings, glutes, back extensors, upper back, and rear shoulder muscles. It also prepares you for more intense back work in poses like Bow and Camel.

Getting into the pose: From Downward Facing Dog, bring your knees and upper body to the floor. Lie facedown and turn one cheek to the floor with your arms to your sides. Reach with your toes and activate your inner thighs and core center, lifting your belly button to your spine. Reach your shoulder blades toward your spine, lifting your chest and shoulders away from your mat, and let your head follow. Keep your palms facing inward and reach your fingers toward your feet.

Holding the pose: Maintain a good connection through your core center to protect your lower back. Imagine that you are stretched like a hammock and continue to reach your toes and head away, spreading the work throughout your body.

Modifications: For less sensation, bring your hands back to the floor under your shoulders, as in Cobra, for more support. For more sensation, lift your legs away from the floor, keeping your feet together.

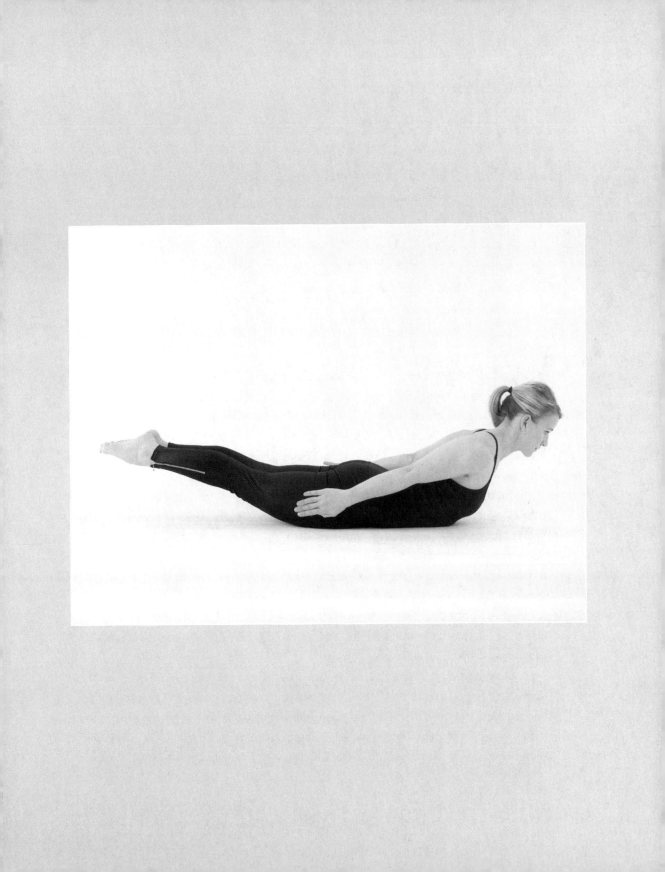

Football/Soccer

Football and soccer demand bursts of explosive, intense speed and also multi-directional movement; they combine sprinting forward, pivoting sideways, turning, leaping, and even squatting to duck. With all those demands, there is all the more reason to keep your body supple and responsive. Stiffness or lack of range of motion are serious liabilities in these sports, and the poses I prescribe here will help to keep your body balanced in strength, mobility, and readiness for the field.

In football, the demands of each position vary drastically, but at any given time an offensive player may be called on to play a defensive role and vice versa. In many of the sports we are covering, you will notice that multiple injuries occur when there is a quick change of direction. A controlled deceleration to a powerful directional change requires alignment and a perfect point of balance to ensure movements are both strong and accurate. Yoga will help you develop the strength to meet these needs.

Players who are generally bigger in stature and rely on their brute strength are still also required to be agile and mobile. Leveraging yoga postures to develop balance and mobility is key for these players.

Football position players such as running backs and receivers rely heavily on their speed, agility, and quickness. If this describes you, my yoga poses will give you the rest and recovery you need and will help hone your mindful alignment; slowing movement patterns to a controlled tempo increases body awareness. The result is precision in movement, which is essential to these athletes.

Quarterbacks, by dint of a repetitive single-arm throw, can have tightness through the chest and often an imbalance of strength and flexibility. A tight or restricted chest and shoulder can hinder the ability to pull back and lengthen yardage gain. All of the poses that encourage chest opening will benefit a quarterback.

In soccer or football, if the field or landscape is uneven, soft, hard, or in any way unpredictable, practicing yoga barefoot will help ensure that the small muscles of the feet and the supportive structure of the ankles are conditioned and responsive to ensure balance and foundation for agility.

Soccer is a game of speed and agility, as well as harnessing different tempos, ranging from explosiveness to contained foot speed. In such a cardio-demanding sport, breath control becomes an integral part of your performance. Quick recoveries and high-intensity plays are more manageable when you are able to control your breath. In a sport where running and impact are unavoidable, the benefits of inversion yoga poses, like Downward Facing Dog, can help alleviate some of the inevitable spinal compression and will lengthen your hamstrings to boot.

In both football and soccer, you'll change directions on a dime quite frequently. Being flexible in your hips will allow you to rely on one leg to hold your body stable, while the other opens up the hip and changes direction. In addition, proper hip mobility ensures efficient movement patterns and can eliminate extra steps and time. Warrior, Side Angle, and Twisting Lunge provide hip opening and strength simultaneously, providing range of motion and stability.

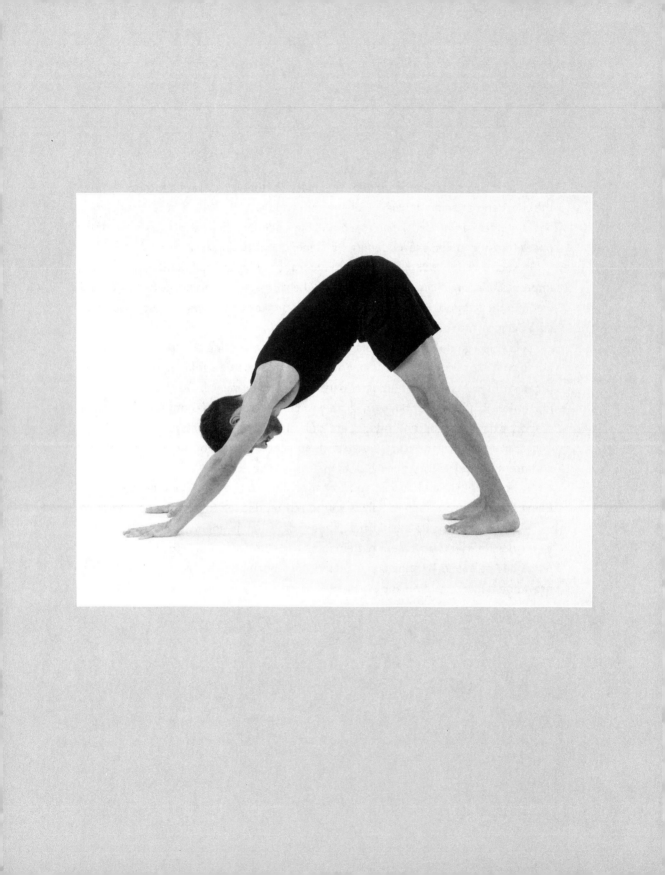

DOWNWARD FACING DOG

Benefit of the pose: This pose opens you across your chest and helps you breathe fully through your abdomen. It opens the front of your shoulders while building shoulder strength. It stretches the whole back of your body, including calves, hamstrings, glutes, and major back muscles. This pose releases tension in the body and, through the inversion effect, aids blood flow to your brain. It creates a sense of alertness to prepare you for what comes next. With regular practice this pose can also be very restful.

Getting into the pose: From Child's Pose, tuck your toes under and reach your arms ahead. Press into your toes and spread your fingers wide while you lift your hips to the sky. Make an inverted V shape with your body.

Holding the pose: Inhale to reach your tailbone up and lengthen your spine. Exhale to bring your chest and belly toward your thighs.

Modifications: If you have a hard time keeping your spine from rounding, bend your knees to keep your hips hinged and your spine long. To relieve tension in your wrists, come down onto the forearms with your elbows shoulder-width apart. Child's Pose is also an option for a rest at any time.

WARRIOR I/WARRIOR LUNGE

Benefit of the pose: This pose opens up the front of your hips on one side while strengthening your hip and thigh muscles on the other. Upper back muscles are also strengthened by staying lifted through the heart. Warrior poses help to keep our hips mobile and strong.

Getting into the pose: From a standing position, step back with one foot and extend your arms above with your shoulders back and down. For Warrior I, lower your back heel to the floor, keeping your pelvis facing forward. For Warrior Lunge, keep your back heel lifted.

Holding the pose: In Warrior I, straighten your back leg and keep all four corners of your back foot on your mat. Feel the work in your pelvis. In Warrior Lunge, keep your front knee over your ankle and press through your back heel to open your hip.

Modifications: If you feel tension in your lower back in Warrior I, lift your heel into Warrior Lunge or step wider side to side to make room to move your pelvis. For less sensation in Warrior Lunge, take your back knee to the floor and place your hands on your front thigh.

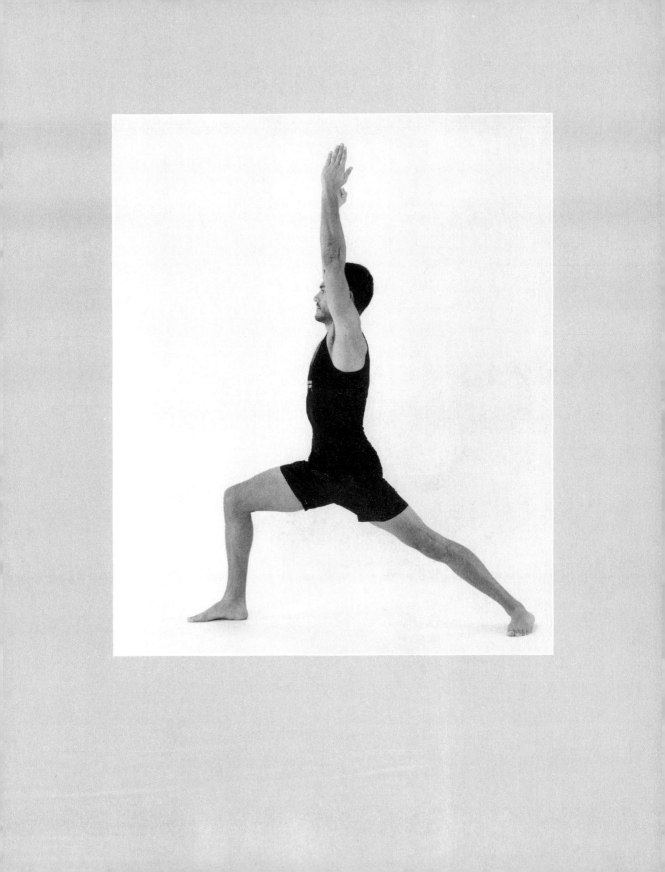

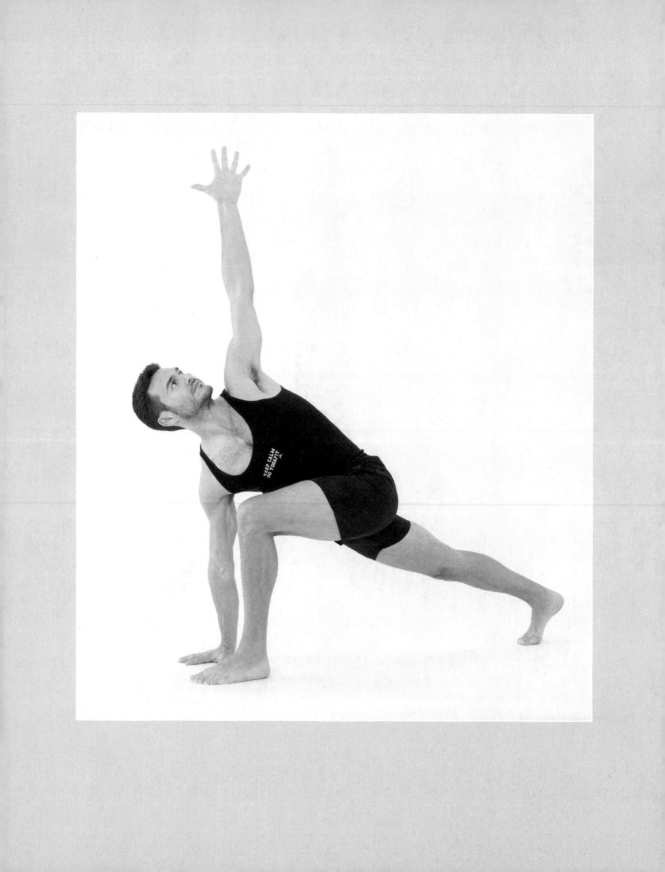

TWISTING LUNGE

Benefit of the pose: Like Warrior Lunge, this pose opens the front of your hips and strengthens your knees, quads, and upper back. The twist strengthens your hip adductors and obliques on one side while stretching them on the opposite side. The twist invigorates your muscles through your whole torso, stimulating conductivity of your sensory nerves and massaging your internal organs.

Getting into the pose: From a Warrior Lunge, lengthen through the crown of your head and keep your spine long. Engage your core center and twist first with your navel, then your chest, then your shoulders toward your front leg.

Holding the pose: Keep one hand on the floor for support and lift the other to the sky. For more sensation, bring your lower arm across your front thigh and bring both hands to your heart. Continue to lengthen your spine, rotate further, and press into your back heel to deepen the posture.

Modifications: You can perform this posture with your back knee down on the mat—with extra padding under your knee for more comfort. You may also place your floor hand on a block for support, which may help to extend your spine.

SIDE ANGLE

Benefit of the pose: In Side Angle you are in the opposite direction of a Twisting Lunge. It works to stabilize your knee while creating mobility in your hips using your hip rotator muscles. We strengthen the muscles in your torso for stability and rotation. This pose also opens your chest and shoulders.

Getting into the pose: From Twisting Lunge, revolve your body open in the opposite direction. As you rotate open, release your back heel to the ground and keep your front knee above your ankle. Place your forearm on the same side as your front leg on your front thigh or your hand to the floor.

Holding the pose: Lift out of your bottom shoulder and reach your opposite hand to the sky with a slight rotation to open your chest and shoulders. Bring the inner thigh of your back leg toward the heel of your front foot to lower your hips.

Modifications: For more support, use a block under your bottom hand to lift through your torso to build torso and core strength. To reduce intensity, bring your top hand to your pelvis.

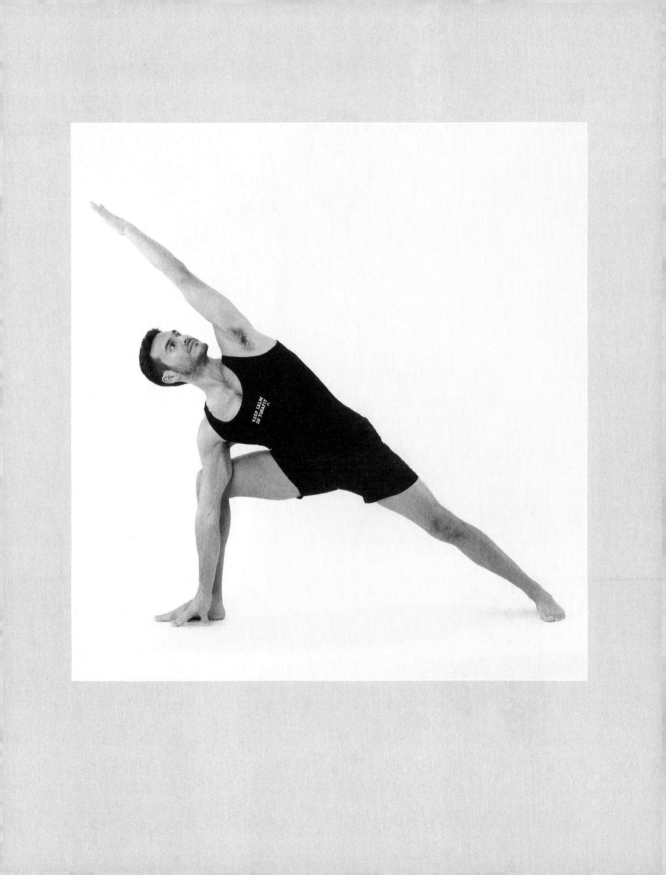

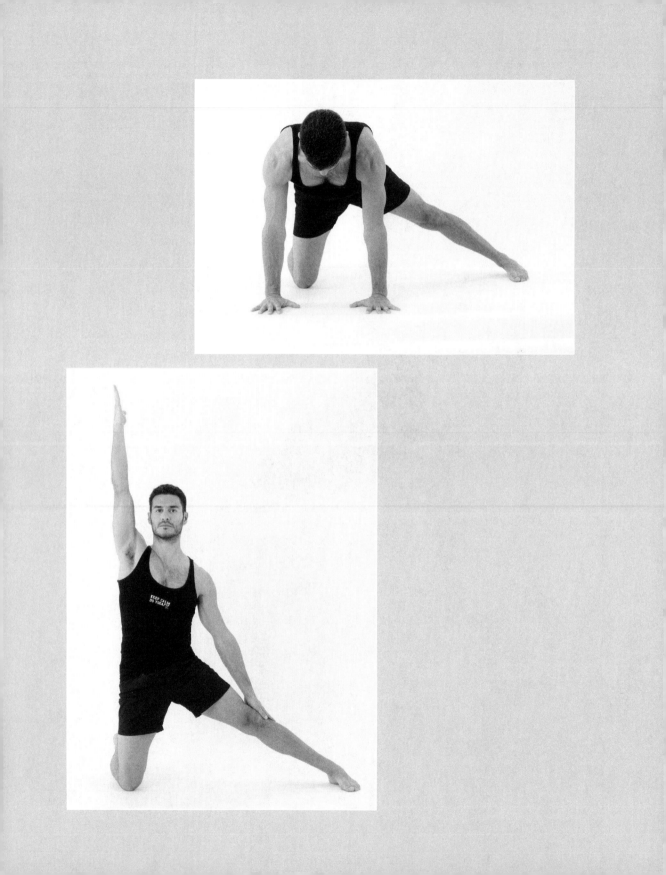

GATE (WITH CAT/COW)

Benefit of the pose: This pose stretches your obliques, inner thighs, and some of the muscles in your back and the outside of your ankle. It also strengthens your torso, legs, and hip stabilizers.

Getting into the pose: From all fours, extend one leg back, pressing through your heel. Keep your leg long and lifted and bring it out to the side. With control, place your foot flat on the ground, toes facing forward. Walk your hands inward and lift your body upward. Raise your arm on the same side as your kneeling leg to open the side of your torso. Place your other hand at your hip or reach out along your extended leg.

Holding the pose: Reach to the sky with your hand, feeling a long line extending through your knee, hip, shoulder, and hand. Reach your extended leg farther from your body, opening your hips and further stretching your inner thighs. Pull your shoulders back and move your hips forward to stay open through your hips and chest.

Option to flow with Cat/Cow: From all fours, we have the option to flow through spinal flexion (Cat) and extension (Cow). Inhale to open your heart forward into Cow, and lift your gaze and tailbone to the sky. Exhale and round your spine like a cat and release your tailbone and your head down. Keep your shoulders back and down. This flow will increase the sensation through the inner thigh of your extended leg.

Modifications: For comfort on the knee, an extra fold in the mat will provide more cushioning. If more hip support is required, come into the pose from kneeling upright and extend one leg to the side.

PIGEON

Benefit of the pose: Great for releasing tension and stress, Pigeon stretches the deep glute muscles in the back of the hips. It also helps to stretch the band of muscle that runs down the outside of the thigh from the hip to the knee that gets tight with a lot of running (IT Band).

Getting into the pose: From Downward Facing Dog, bring one leg forward to the floor with your knee bent and your foot flexed. Stay lifted enough to keep your pelvis level.

Holding the pose: Release your upper body down to the floor and rest your forehead on your hands or stacked fists.

Modifications: To make this pose more restorative, lie on your back with your knees bent and your feet on the floor. Lift one leg and place your foot on your other thigh for support. Reach to hold the supporting leg behind the knee and draw your leg in toward your chest. If your range of motion allows, Standing Pigeon from Chair Pose is another option. Bring one ankle to the top of the opposite thigh with your foot flexed and sit back into Chair Pose.

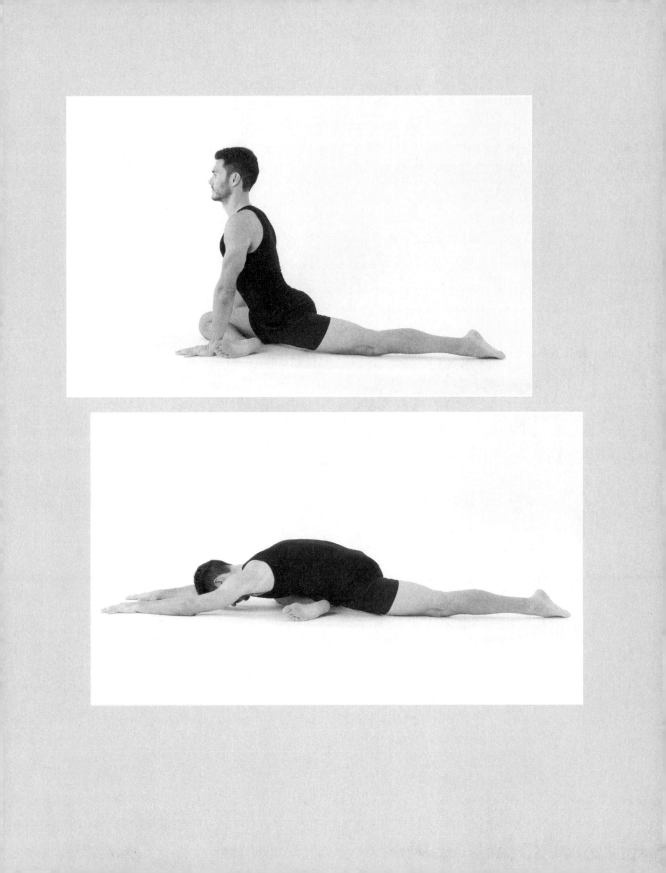

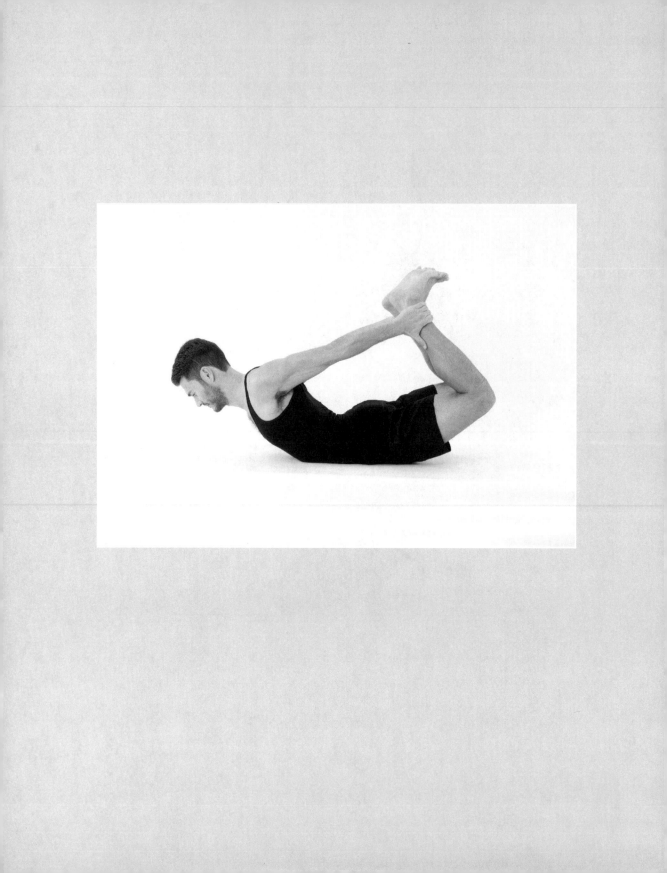

BOW

Benefit of the pose: Bow opens up the whole front side of the body—quads, hip flexors, abdominals, chest, and shoulders—while strengthening the entire back side of the body, including your hamstrings, glutes, back extensors, and upper back. Performed with intense levels of exertion, it helps the body to release tension and pent-up energy. This pose is great for offsetting excessive amounts of forward flexion (rounding of the spine and shoulders).

Getting into the pose: Lie on your belly and open your shoulders to reach behind to your ankles. Flex your feet and draw your thighs inward. Press your ankles into your hands and hold your ankles firmly. Engage your core center and lift away from the body.

Holding the pose: Keep a strong core center and continue to lift through the crown of your head and press your ankles into your hands.

Modifications: If you have difficulty getting both hands to your ankles, use Half Bow, which is performed one side at a time. Place one arm in front of you bent at the elbow. Use your hand and forearm across your mat for support and reach your other hand to the ankle on the same side. Another option is to place a strap around your ankle and hold on to the strap.

Golf/Tennis

Golf and tennis favor one side of the body. Your handedness determines that strength. If you're a tennis player, you are likely stronger on your forehand side. Golfers are almost always stronger in their bottom grip arm and their planted foot leg. That's natural—you are using the muscles on your forehand or driving swing side more than those on your backhand or nonswing side.

Of course, in tennis, you can work on your backhand and strengthen both forearms and quads to support great swings from either side. But then there's also your serve, which uses your forehand arm and shoulder to power the ball over the net. No matter how much you work on that backhand, you're still going to use your forehand more when you add in your serves, meaning you favor that forehand side.

Tennis is a game of multiple plane movements, and the intensity to gain position prior to executing a racquet swing requires a high level of agility, speed, balance, stability, coordination, and power.

The demands of both the forehand and backhand strokes involve rotational force, controlled racquet position, angle, and follow-through. Yoga will allow you to strengthen stability and balance while slowing the tempo of rotation for mindful muscle recruitment. Repeating these movements slowly in yoga allows for precision and an earned progression in tempo while on the court. Alignment of your ball strike begins with getting in proper position, and on some shots the ability to execute a shot while off-balance is a requirement as well. Given the dynamic nature of the sport, rest, regeneration, and recovery through yoga is essential.

Golf is the only sport where taking fewer shots is the desired outcome. This of course means that it is every golfer's quest to achieve the best possible shot in every attempt. A combination of strength and accuracy is required for longer drives, while great body control and awareness are necessary for the shorter game. One of the challenges of the game is the constant need to adapt to varying surfaces while still being able to execute a smooth and accurate club swing. A heightened awareness of body position, alignment, and weight transfer will prove to add accuracy to your shot and subtract strokes from your scorecard.

While executing a proper golf swing, multiple muscles are engaged to activate a cross-body movement sequence. The rotating movement requires great range of motion as the body extends or uncoils and contracts or coils to generate head speed. Ensuring controlled movement through the full range of motion of a swing will provide accuracy and desired ball play. Balance and stability serves as a foundation to initiate control through the backswing, accuracy of ball strike, and proper follow-through to provide the best shot possible.

Grip strength through the fingers prevents the club from spinning or slipping in one's hands. This is true for any sport that uses a racquet, stick, or club. Postures that include flexion, extension, and rotation of the wrists help with range of motion and stability.

In both golf and tennis, a mindful calmness and controlled breathing permit the body and mind to fully prepare for an accurate shot. A controlled breathing sequence of an inhale on the backswing and an exhale on the swing in play will improve your swing every time.

Due to the necessary asymmetrical movement, many golfers and tennis players find that their pelvis becomes tilted or offset, leading to strain on the lower back, tightness in the hips, and poor knee alignment. When there is an imbalance or misalignment of the hips or pelvis, the body responds by trying to straighten it, leading to tightness on one side and strain on the other. These imbalances can lead to pain and injury. My YogaFit poses help to create length in both sides of your body and promote strength and mobility in your shoulders and hips. In other words, these poses will develop stability and power for a more effective swing.

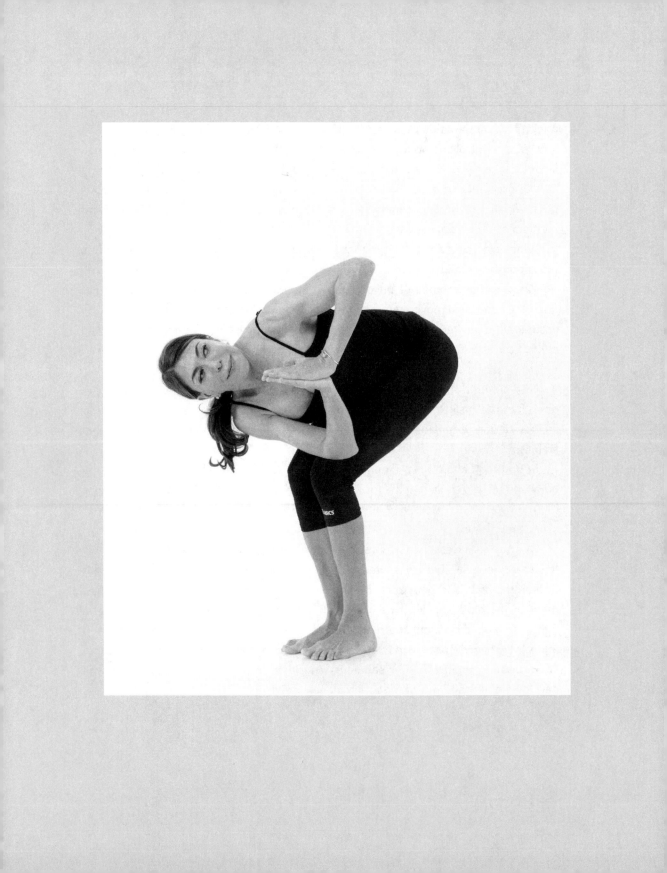

REVOLVING CHAIR

Benefit of the pose: Much like Chair, this strengthens your hips, quads, and upper torso. It also strengthens your obliques and stretches your lower back. The twist invigorates your torso muscles, stimulates conductivity of your sensory nerves, and massages your internal organs. Revolving Chair also trains torso rotation with open chest and shoulders, which you need for an effective tennis or golf swing. It stretches the glutes as well, which work to generate a lot of power in a swing.

Getting into the pose: From a standing position, bring your feet and legs together and sit back into Chair Pose with your hands together at your heart. From Chair, keep your legs and feet together and twist first from your navel, then your chest, then your shoulders. Once in the twist, you may also open up your arms and reach to the floor and sky.

Holding the pose: Breathe in to lengthen your spine and breathe out to rotate further. Keep your knees level with each other. As you reach your arm to the sky, pull the shoulder blade on the same side toward your spine to open your chest. Engage your core center to support your spine.

Modifications: For less sensation and more support, bring the arm on the side you are twisting toward onto your lower back. Gently reach across and place your other hand on the opposite thigh.

STANDING HAND-to-LEG BALANCE with TWIST

Benefit of the pose: Balance and posture improve with this pose. It also strengthens the glutes and hamstrings of your standing leg and upper back muscles to stand tall. For your raised leg, it brings your femur into your hip joint and stretches your hamstring.

Getting into the pose: Stand on one leg and lift the opposite leg, starting with a bent knee. Extend your raised leg in front of you. Stand tall and keep your standing leg long and your hip extended and engage your core center. Extend your raised leg while holding on to your foot or toe or use a strap. For the twist, inhale and lengthen your spine and reach the opposite hand to your raised foot, allowing your other arm to reach back, twisting first from your navel, then your chest, then your shoulders.

Holding the pose: Focus on standing tall to work your hamstrings, glutes, and back muscles. Inhale and lengthen your spine and exhale to rotate further or focus on holding for strength.

Modifications: If your spine rounds, bend your raised leg so that you can stand straight. Hold your raised leg bent 90 degrees at the knee and resting your foot on a chair or bench. You may also use a strap around the foot of your extended leg so that you don't have to reach as far to your foot.

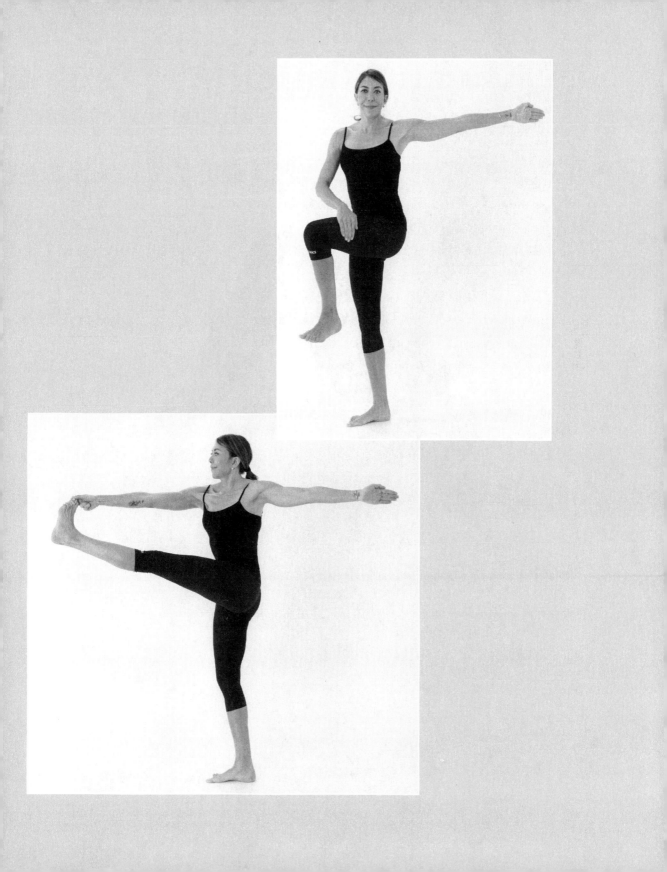

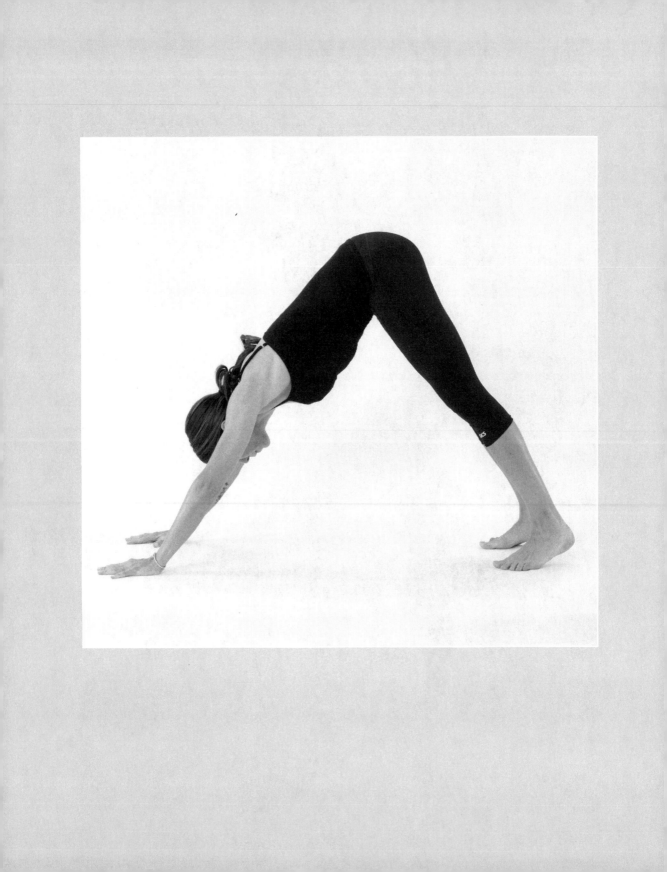

DOWNWARD FACING DOG

Benefit of the pose: This pose opens you across your chest and helps you breathe fully through your abdomen. It opens the front of your shoulders while building shoulder strength. It stretches the whole back of your body, including calves, hamstrings, glutes, and major back muscles. This pose releases tension in the body and, through the inversion effect, aids blood flow to your brain. It creates a sense of alertness to prepare you for what comes next. With regular practice this pose can also be very restful.

Getting into the pose: From Child's Pose, tuck your toes under and reach your arms ahead. Press into your toes and spread your fingers wide while you lift your hips to the sky. Make an inverted V shape with your body.

Holding the pose: Inhale to reach your tailbone up and lengthen your spine. Exhale to bring your chest and belly toward your thighs.

Modifications: If you have a hard time keeping your spine from rounding, bend your knees to keep your hips hinged and your spine long. To relieve tension in your wrists, come down onto the forearms with your elbows shoulder-width apart. Child's Pose is also an option for a rest at any time.

SPINAL BALANCE

Benefit of the pose: Spinal Balance encourages your core center muscles to stabilize as you resist gravity. It also strengthens your glutes, upper and lower back, chest, and shoulders.

Getting into the pose: From your hands and knees, stabilize your shoulders and hips. Extend one arm out at the height of your shoulder. Lift the opposite leg just to the height of your hips.

Holding the pose: Keep a long line from your fingers to your heel and hold for 5–10 breaths. Focus on stability and strength while you lift your navel to your spine. You may also flow this pose: Inhale as you lengthen your arm and leg and exhale as you bring them back to the floor, then switch sides. Continue to reach forward with your fingers and press back through your heel, toes to the floor, with little or no movement in the torso. Repeat 5–10 times per side.

Modifications: To relieve wrist tension, use fists for wrists, palms facing each other. For knee comfort, place padding or make a fold in the mat to kneel on. For less sensation, extend just the arm or just the leg.

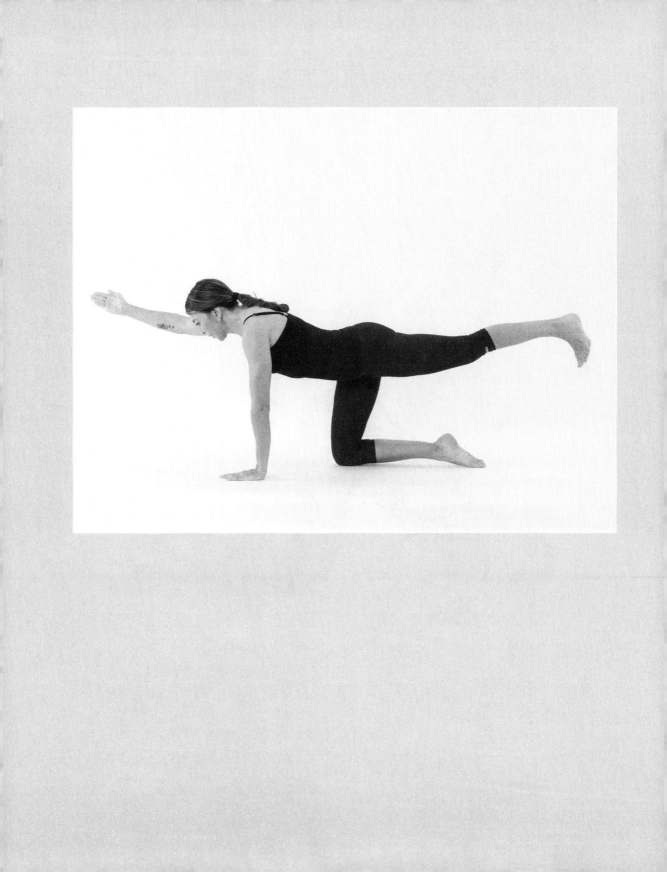

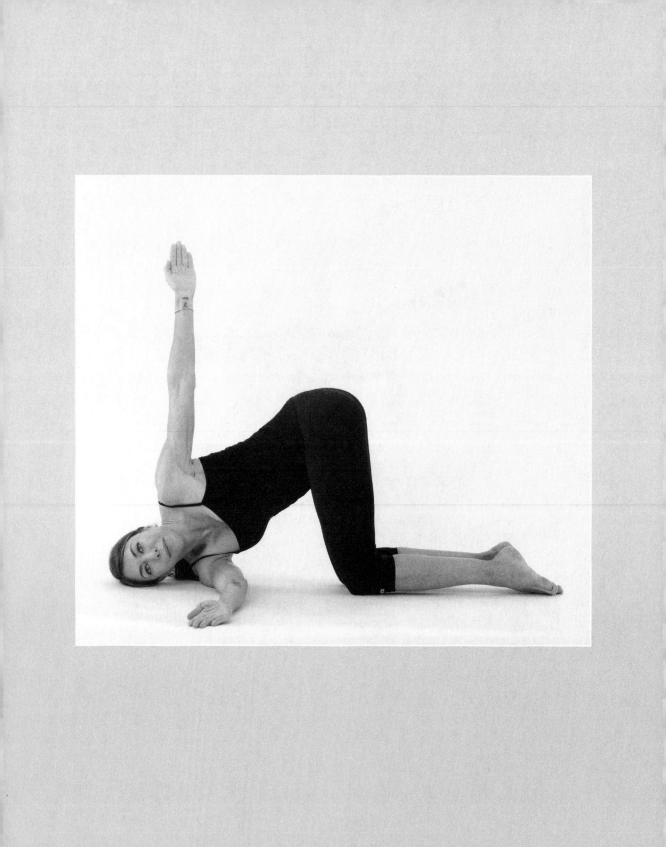

THREAD the NEEDLE

Benefit of the pose: This posture stretches your lower back and chest and the rear of one shoulder and the front of the other shoulder. With your head down and your hips up, your spine is not compressed by gravity in this rotation. It reinforces spinal alignment and length across your shoulders through a rotation as well.

Getting into the pose: From all fours, lift one arm forward with your thumb to the sky. Then bring your arm through the space between your opposite arm and your leg. As you twist, keep your pelvis level and above the knees. Engage through your core center to support your spine and your lower back through rotation. Flow with breath for movement in your upper spine or hold to deepen the stretch.

Holding the pose: Keep your pelvis above the knees, and if you feel supported enough, lift your upper arm to the sky or rest your hand on your hip or lower back. To hold this pose, rest your upper body on the mat for a stretch to the outside of your shoulder. To flow, inhale as you lift your lower arm out and upward, reaching away from the floor. Exhale to lower down into the twist and continue to move with your breath.

Modifications: For knee comfort, place padding or make a fold in the mat to kneel on. Leave the opposite arm on the floor for support. You may also have a soft block under your head for comfort or bring your raised hand back to the floor.

LOCUST

Benefit of the pose: This pose strengthens the entire back of the body, including your hamstrings, glutes, back extensors, upper back, and rear shoulder muscles. It also prepares you for more intense back work in poses like Bow and Camel.

Getting into the pose: Lie facedown and turn one cheek to the floor with your arms to your sides. Reach with your toes and activate your inner thighs and core center, lifting your belly button to your spine. Reach your shoulder blades toward your spine, lifting your chest and shoulders away from your mat, and let your head follow. Keep your palms facing inward and reach your fingers toward your feet.

Holding the pose: Maintain a good connection through your core center to protect your lower back. Imagine that you are stretched like a hammock and continue to reach your toes and head away, spreading the work throughout your body.

Modifications: For less sensation, bring your hands back to the floor under your shoulders, as in Cobra, for more support. For more sensation, lift your legs away from the floor, keeping your feet together.

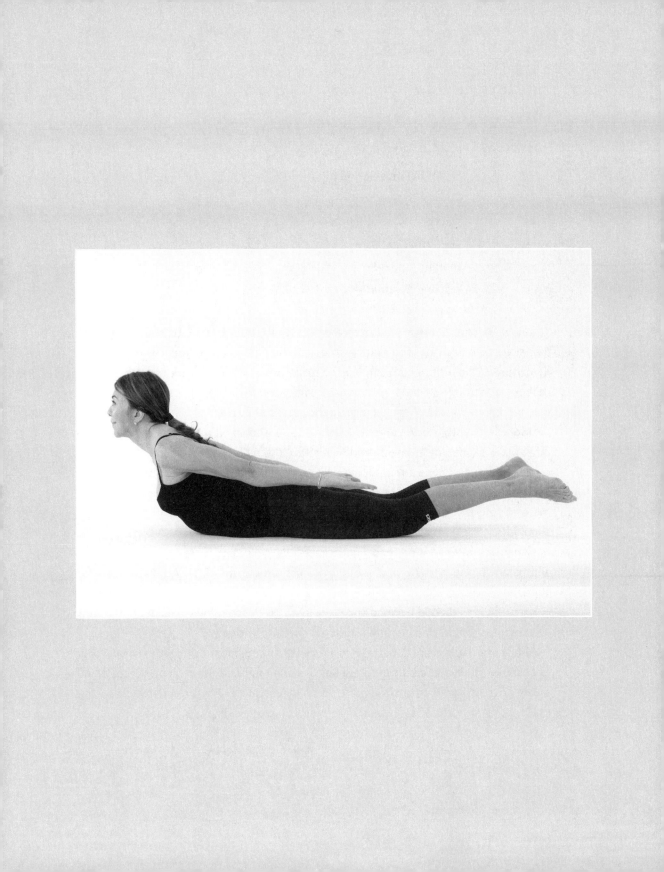

Hockey

Hockey players are on the icefor short but intense periods of time in which they skate hard and fast. The skating stride and high intensity on the ice create a lot of demands on the hips, which can lead to groin injuries, so we want to keep the hips mobile and strong. We must also consider the need for balance, rotation, and shoulder stability—all needed when shooting the puck.

More frequently, hockey injuries occur due to impact with the boards, the ice, or other players; shoulders, knees, and heads take the most impact. For this reason you want to build total body strength and control while keeping your mind and body alert and responsive. Overall, to perform well and reduce injuries, these yoga poses promote alertness and body awareness as well as facilitating mobility in the hips and shoulders.

When you are shooting, passing, or receiving passes, you are typically in motion and balancing on one leg or the other the majority of the time. And when you are checking—loading and unloading your weight as you gain position and prepare for impact—you need good balance and stability to produce an effective check. Shooting also requires weight transfer and rotational strength and power.

While skating, you are constantly in a forward flex position, calling for a strong back or posterior chain and a strong core. Hips are often tight, limiting range of motion for pivots or transitioning from backward to forward skating. Any inversion poses—like

Downward Facing Dog—will feel wonderful, taking compression off of your lower back.

The Warrior poses assist in hip opening and strength, training alignment and breath control. Hockey players will also enjoy the benefits of balance through Triangle and Twisting Pyramid. In these two poses the major requirements of balance, rotation, and forward flexion are addressed through lengthening, opening, and stability.

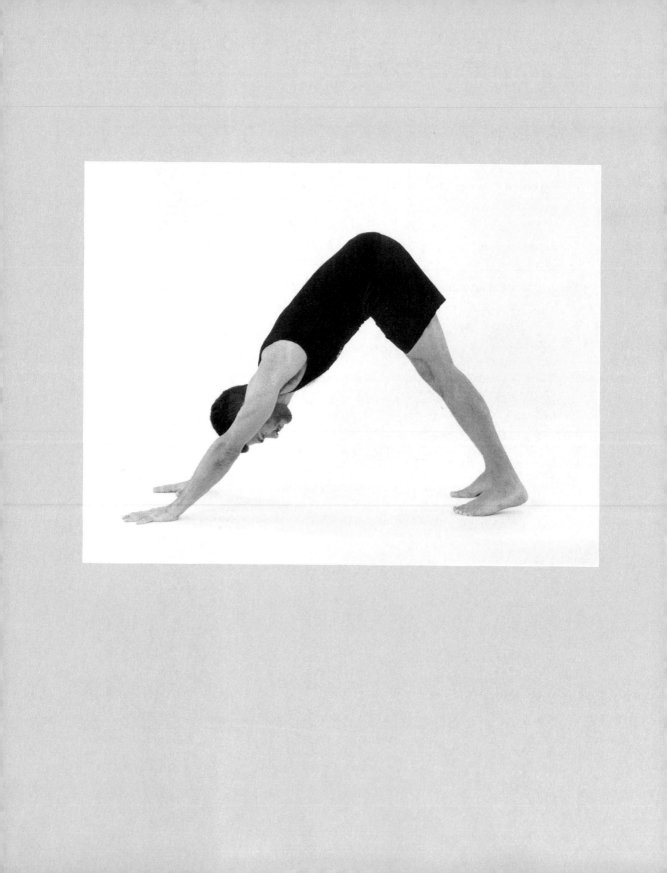

DOWNWARD FACING DOG

Benefit of the pose: This pose opens you across your chest and helps you breathe fully through your abdomen. It opens the front of your shoulders while building shoulder strength. It stretches the whole back of your body, including calves, hamstrings, glutes, and major back muscles. This pose releases tension in the body and, through the inversion effect, aids blood flow to your brain. It creates a sense of alertness to prepare you for what comes next. With regular practice this pose can also be very restful.

Getting into the pose: From Child's Pose, tuck your toes under and reach your arms ahead. Press into your toes and spread your fingers wide while you lift your hips to the sky. Make an inverted V shape with your body.

Holding the pose: Inhale to reach your tailbone up and lengthen your spine. Exhale to bring your chest and belly toward your thighs.

Modifications: If you have a hard time keeping your spine from rounding, bend your knees to keep your hips hinged and your spine long. To relieve tension in your wrists, come down onto the forearms with your elbows shoulder-width apart. Child's Pose is also an option for a rest at any time.

SPINAL BALANCE

Benefit of the pose: Spinal Balance encourages your core center muscles to stabilize as you resist gravity. It also strengthens your glutes, upper and lower back, chest, and shoulders.

Getting into the pose: From your hands and knees, stabilize your shoulders and hips. Extend one arm out at the height of your shoulder. Lift the opposite leg just to the height of your hips.

Holding the pose: Keep a long line from your fingers to your heel and hold for 5–10 breaths. Focus on stability and strength while you lift your navel to your spine. You may also flow this pose: Inhale as you lengthen your arm and leg and exhale as you bring them back to the floor, then switch sides. Continue to reach forward with your fingers and press back through your heel, toes to the floor, with little or no movement in the torso. Repeat 5–10 times per side.

Modifications: To relieve wrist tension, use fists for wrists, palms facing each other. For knee comfort, place padding or make a fold in the mat to kneel on. For less sensation, extend just the arm or just the leg.

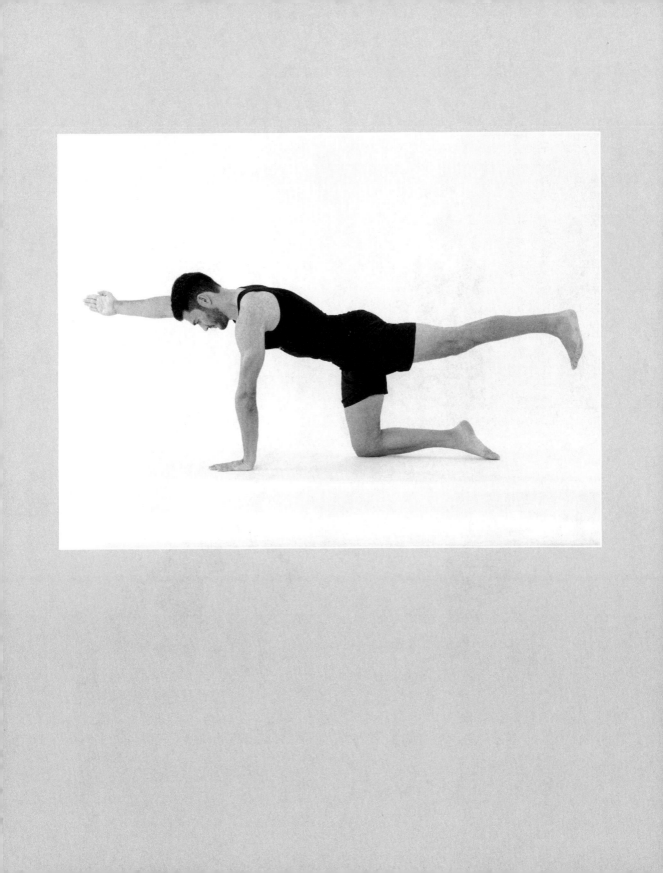

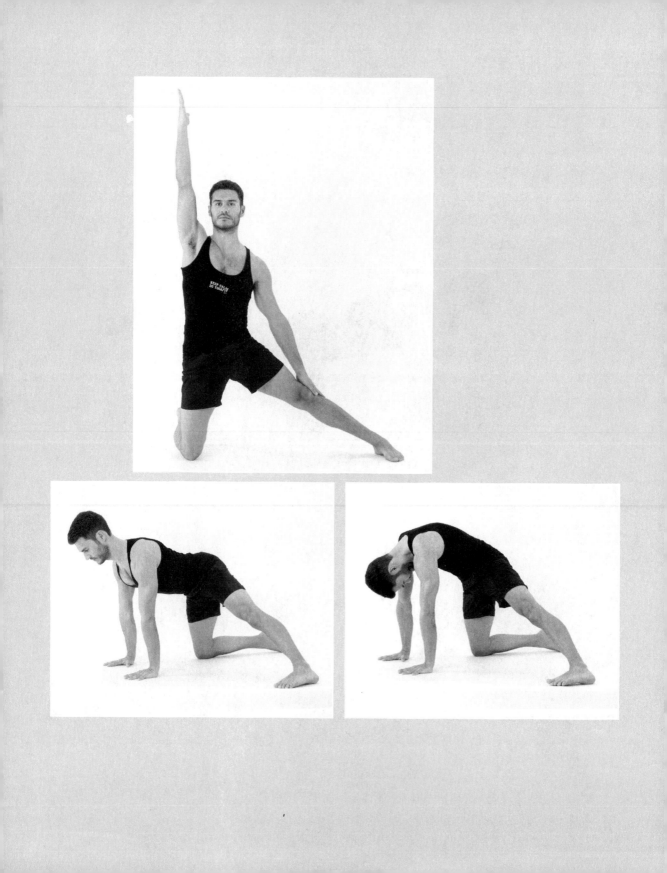

GATE (WITH CAT / COW)

Benefit of the pose: This pose stretches your obliques, inner thighs, and some of the muscles in your back and the outside of your ankle. It also strengthens your torso, legs, and hip stabilizers.

Getting into the pose: From all fours, extend one leg back, pressing through your heel. Keep your leg long and lifted and bring it out to the side. With control, place your foot flat on the ground, toes facing forward. Walk your hands inward and lift your body upward. Raise the arm on the same side as your kneeling leg to open the side of your torso. Place your other hand at your hip or reach out along your extended leg.

Holding the pose: Reach to the sky with your hand, feeling a long line extending through your knee, hip, shoulder, and hand. Reach your extended leg farther from your body, opening your hips and further stretching your inner thighs. Pull your shoulders back and move your hips forward to stay open through your hips and chest.

Option to flow with Cat/Cow: From all fours, we have the option to flow through spinal flexion (Cat) and extension (Cow). Inhale to open your heart forward into Cow, and lift your gaze and tailbone to the sky. Exhale and round your spine like a cat and release your tailbone and head down. Keep your shoulders back and down. This flow will increase the sensation through your inner thigh of your extended leg.

Modifications: For comfort on the knee, an extra fold in the mat will provide more cushioning. If more hip support is required, come into the pose from kneeling upright and extend one leg to the side.

WARRIOR I/WARRIOR LUNGE

Benefit of the pose: This pose opens up the front of your hips on one side while strengthening your hip and thigh muscles on the other. Upper back muscles are also strengthened by staying lifted through the heart. Warrior poses help to keep our hips mobile and strong.

Getting into the pose: From a standing position, step back with one foot and extend your arms above with your shoulders back and down. For Warrior I, lower your back heel to the floor, keeping your pelvis facing forward. For Warrior Lunge, keep your back heel lifted.

Holding the pose: In Warrior I, straighten your back leg and keep all four corners of your back foot on your mat. Feel the work in your pelvis. In Warrior Lunge, keep your front knee over your ankle and press through your back heel to open your hip.

Modifications: If you feel tension in your lower back in Warrior I, lift your heel into Warrior Lunge or step wider side to side to make room to move your pelvis. For less sensation in Warrior Lunge, take your back knee to the floor and place your hands on your front thigh.

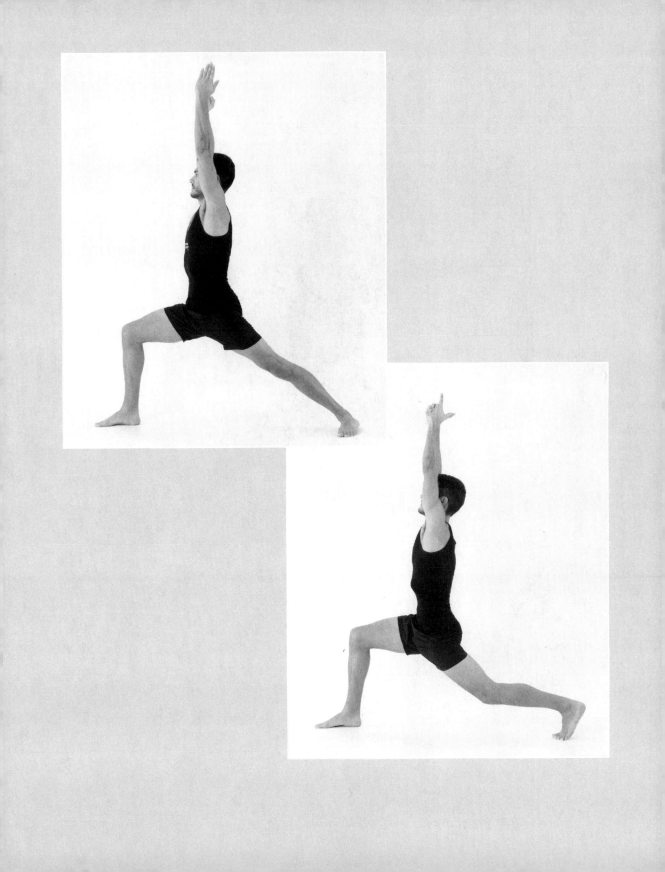

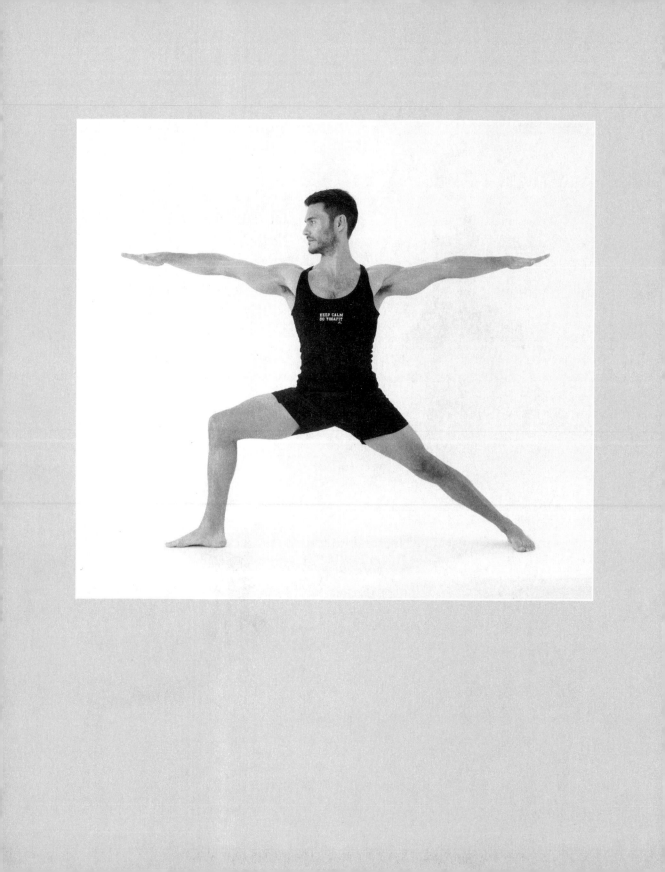

WARRIOR II

Benefit of the pose: Warrior II stretches inner thighs and calves while strengthening the quads, glutes, hamstrings, upper back, and shoulders. It increases your ability to deal with stress and improves your focus.

Getting into the pose: From Warrior I/Warrior Lunge, keep your front knee over the ankle. Inhale and lift your body slightly upward and rotate your torso open to the long edge of your mat. Look over your front fingers as you lower your body.

Holding the pose: Reach forward and back with your arms and keep your pelvis directly beneath your ribs. Continue to notice your knee and make sure it stays over the front ankle. Engage your core center and lift through the top of your head to stay long through your torso. Relax your shoulders back and down.

Modifications: For less intensity, shorten your stance and be up a little higher. To relieve tension in the neck and shoulders bring your hands to your heart.

TRIANGLE

Benefit of the pose: Triangle works with Warrior poses to stretch and strengthen your groin. It targets hamstrings and inner thighs for a great stretch and strengthens your quads, obliques, hip flexors, and rear shoulders.

Getting into the pose: From Warrior II, reach forward with your front arm while you lengthen your front leg with a micro bend in the front knee. Keep the upper side of your body long; the spine does not flex down. Reach your arms to the earth and sky.

Holding the pose: Engage your glutes to bring your pelvis in line with your legs. Rotate your torso upward and continue to reach to the earth and sky and reach through the crown of your head.

Modifications: For less sensation, lower the top hand to your hip. If you are rounding to the floor, place a block under your hand for support. Do this pose against a wall to feel where your hips, shoulders, and head should align.

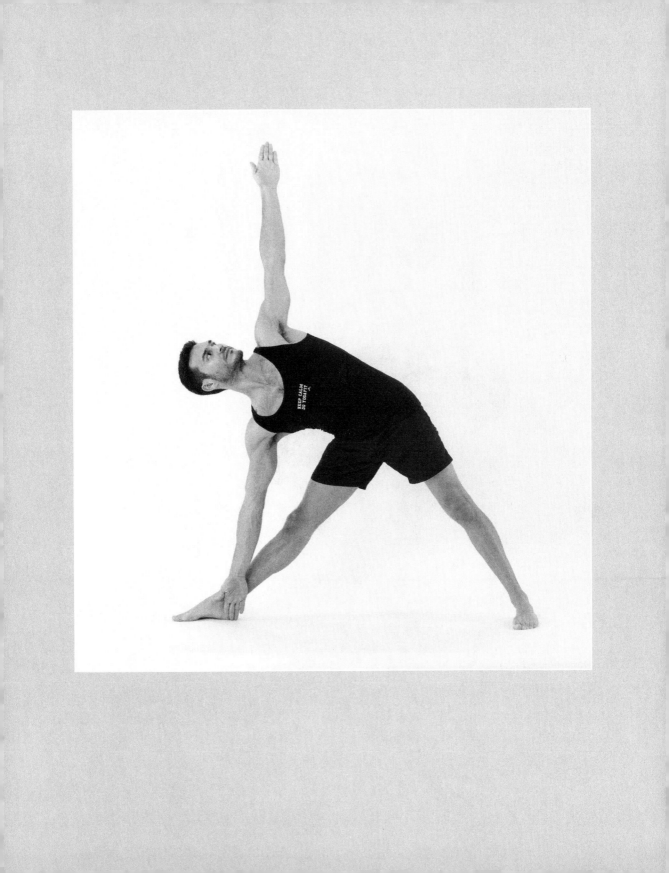

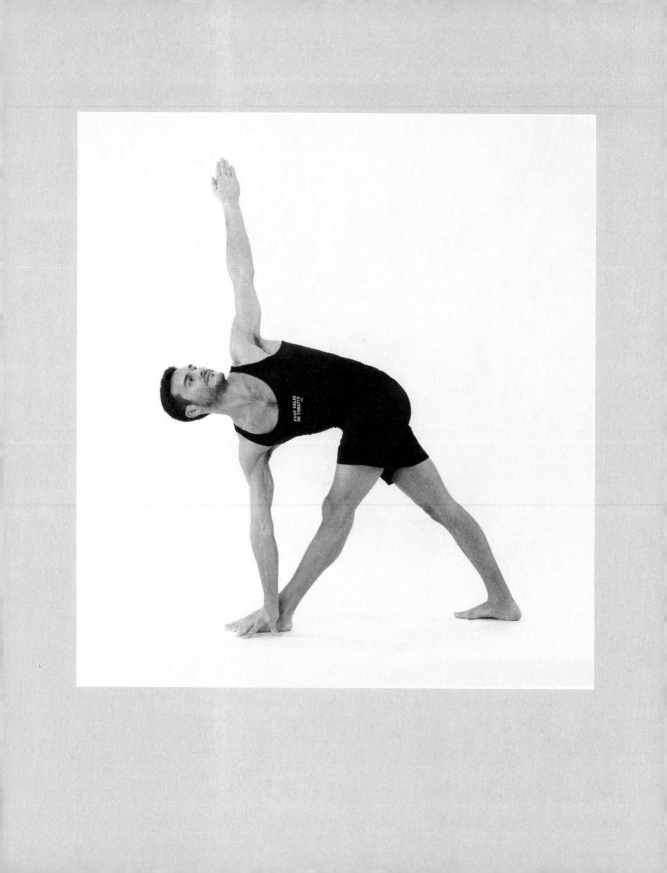

TWISTING PYRAMID

Benefit of the pose: Twisting Pyramid (revolved triangle) stretches your hamstrings, lower back, and the outside and back of your hips and your obliques. It also strengthens your quads, inner thighs, obliques, upper back, and shoulders. It works to offset a lot of hip extension as in skating.

Getting into the pose: From Triangle, turn your body to face the floor and shorten your stance a little. Square your pelvis and keep your spine extended and parallel to the floor. Twist from your navel, then your chest, then your shoulders toward your front leg. Your lower arm can come to the floor or across your front leg while you reach your other arm to the sky.

Holding the pose: Continue to reach toward the sky while you pull the top of your shoulder blade toward your spine. Engage your inner thighs to keep your pelvis level while you reach through the crown of your head.

Modifications: If your hamstrings feel tight, bend your front knee a little. You may also lower your raised arm to your hips. If you are rounding your spine, place a block under your hand for support and to find more lift in the torso.

Running

There are many levels of running—from recreational runs on city streets or trails to half and full marathons, and various track and field events at all levels (from school to Olympics and even professional). Avid runners—people who run often and for long periods or at high speeds—are most susceptible to overuse injuries, but falling on a course can bring about injury too. To defend against either kind of injury, it is important to maintain good running skills with a balanced body. My poses—especially Pigeon—promote that balance. Furthermore, since yoga is done barefoot, these poses promote good foot and ankle health, which are obviously important for runners.

Due to the single-leg impact in the running motion, your body absorbs and stabilizes through the ankle, knee, and hip joints. This often results in tightness in your hamstrings, hips, and glutes. The simple inversion of Downward Facing Dog will lengthen the leg muscles and help take compression off the lower back (exacerbated by the often unforgiving surfaces you run on, like pavement or concrete). The Single Leg Stretch can assist in recovery and muscle balance while Bridge helps strengthen the hamstrings. Pigeon and Twisting Lunge are also great favorites of runners, due to their focus on opening and lengthening the pelvis and hip complex.

Due to the nature of long distance running, breath control and achieving maximum oxygen uptake are important skills; they help you sustain your pace and performance throughout long runs. Awareness of posture—a benefit of these poses—can also impact your ability to breathe properly and execute running techniques that are both effective and efficient.

A regular yoga practice can enhance and ensure muscle balance and strength. Runners who commit to strength and flexibility training can ensure joint stability and alignment so that they can enjoy their sport for a long time and many miles to come.

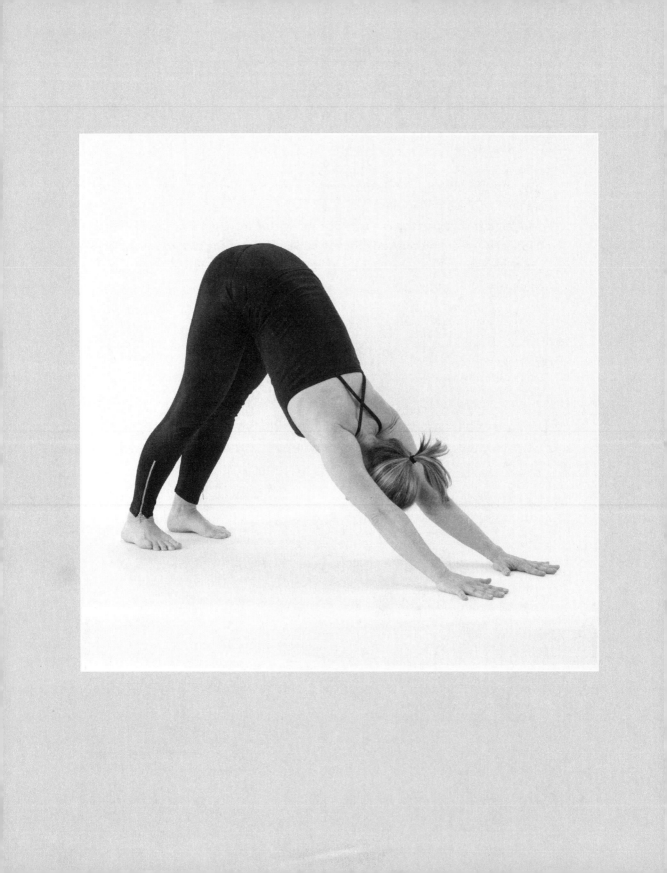

DOWNWARD FACING DOG

Benefit of the pose: This pose opens you across your chest and helps you breathe fully through your abdomen. It opens the front of your shoulders while building shoulder strength. It stretches the whole back of your body, including calves, hamstrings, glutes, and major back muscles. This pose releases tension in the body and, through the inversion effect, aids blood flow to your brain. It creates a sense of alertness to prepare you for what comes next. With regular practice this pose can also be very restful.

Getting into the pose: From Child's Pose, tuck your toes under and reach your arms ahead. Press into your toes and spread your fingers wide while you lift your hips to the sky. Make an inverted V shape with your body.

Holding the pose: Inhale to reach your tailbone up and lengthen your spine. Exhale to bring your chest and belly toward your thighs.

Modifications: If you have a hard time keeping your spine from rounding, bend your knees to keep your hips hinged and your spine long. To relieve tension in your wrists, come down onto the forearms with your elbows shoulder-width apart. Child's Pose is also an option for a rest at any time.

TWISTING LUNGE

Benefit of the pose: Like Warrior Lunge, this pose opens the front of your hips and strengthens your knees, quads, and upper back. The twist strengthens your hip adductors and obliques on one side while stretching them on the opposite side. The twist invigorates the muscles through your whole torso, stimulating conductivity of your sensory nerves and massaging your internal organs.

Getting into the pose: From a Warrior Lunge, lengthen through the crown of your head and keep your spine long. Engage your core center and twist first with your navel, then your chest, then your shoulders toward your front leg.

Holding the pose: Keep one hand on the floor for support and lift the other to the sky. For more sensation, bring your lower arm across your front thigh and bring both hands to your heart. Continue to lengthen your spine, rotate further and press into your back heel to deepen the posture.

Modifications: You can perform this posture with your back knee down on the mat—with extra padding under your knee for more comfort. You may also place your floor hand on a block for support, which may help to extend your spine.

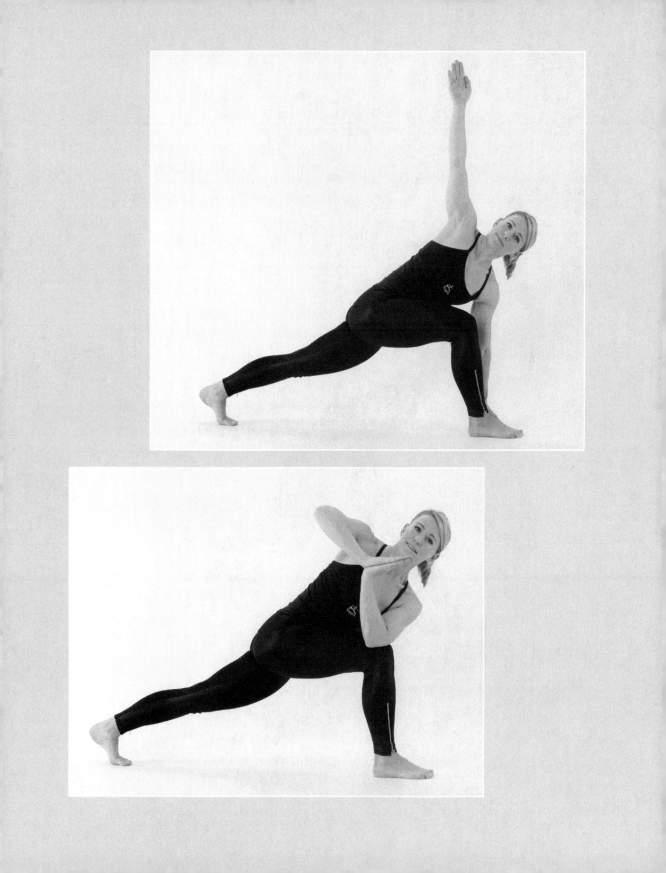

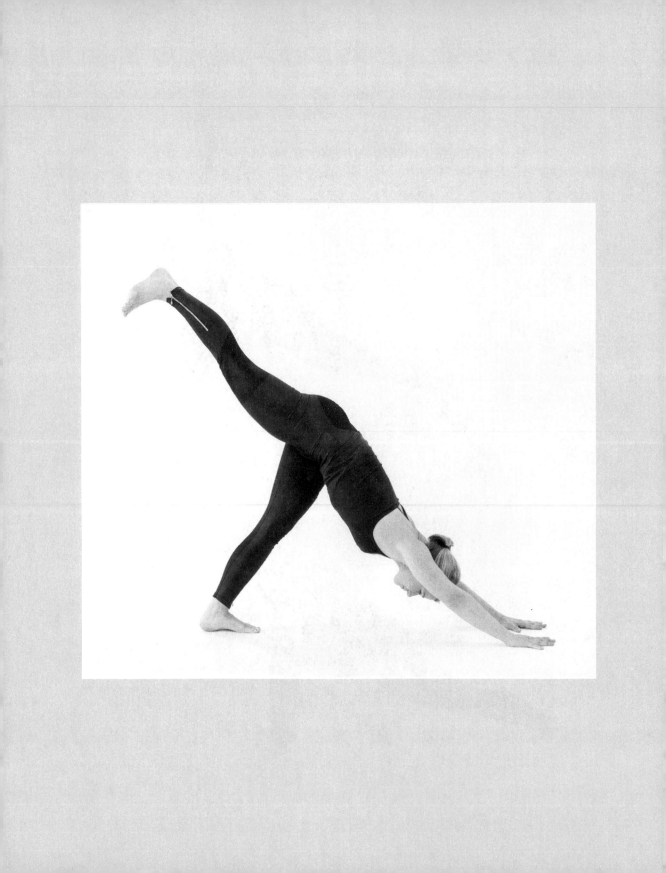

THREE-LEGGED DOG

Benefit of the pose: In addition to the benefits of Downward Facing Dog, this pose allows you to strengthen your glutes and stretch your hip flexors and hip extensors. By lifting one leg, it also builds more shoulder strength with the added weight above.

Getting into the pose: From Downward Facing Dog, extend one leg back and up, keeping it as straight as possible.

Holding the pose: Keep your foot flexed with your toes, knees, and hip facing the floor. Reach long from your hand to your heel.

Modifications: Spinal Balance is a great alternative if this pose is too much for the shoulders for any reason.

TRIPOD DOG

Benefit of the pose: Tripod Dog prepares your hips for Pigeon. It stretches the outer glute and thigh (IT Band) of the leg that is underneath, as well as the outer calf and ankle.

Getting into the pose: From Downward Facing Dog, bring one leg underneath your body and extend it across your mat to the opposite side with your foot flexed.

Holding the pose: Shift your hips away from your hands as in Downward Facing Dog, hinging your hips and keeping your spine long, adding to the stretch on the outside of the leg down along your calf and ankle.

Modifications: If there is a buildup of tension in your hips or down your leg, shift forward to release the tension and enjoy a milder stretch.

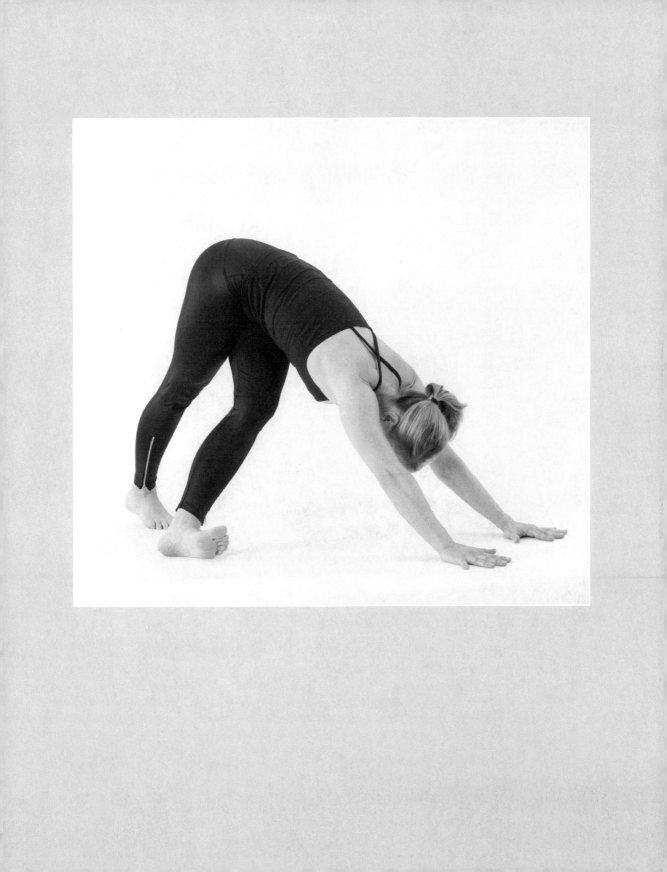

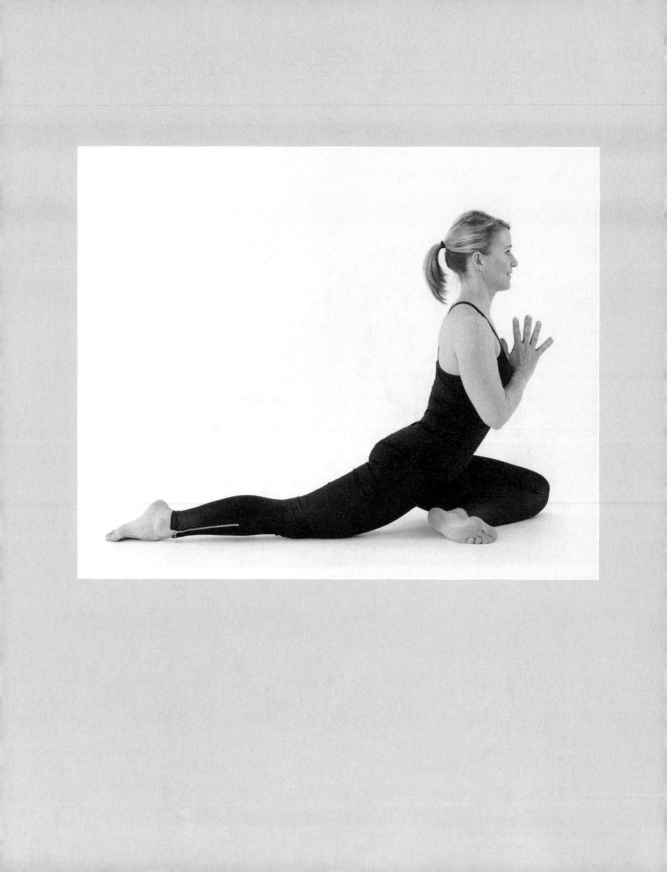

PIGEON

Benefit of the pose: Great for releasing tension and stress, Pigeon stretches the deep glute muscles in the back of the hips. It also helps to stretch the band of muscle that runs down the outside of the thigh from the hip to the knee that gets tight with a lot of running (IT Band).

Getting into the pose: From Downward Facing Dog, bring one leg forward to the floor with your knee bent and your foot flexed. Stay lifted enough to keep your pelvis level. From Tripod Dog, bend your forward leg and lower.

Holding the pose: Release your upper body down to the floor and rest your forehead on your hands or stacked fists.

Modifications: To make this pose more restorative, lie on your back with your knees bent and your feet on the floor. Lift one leg and place your foot on your other thigh for support. Reach to hold the supporting leg behind the knee and draw your leg in toward your chest. If your range of motion allows, Standing Pigeon from Chair Pose is another option. Bring one ankle to the top of the opposite thigh with your foot flexed and sit back into Chair Pose.

SINGLE LEG STRETCH

Benefit of the pose: This pose isolates the hamstrings in a relaxed position. While on the floor you will be able to feel the alignment of your spine along the floor. You will also feel shifting in your pelvis as you stretch one leg.

Getting into the pose: Lie on your back and extend one leg on your mat while lifting your other leg up to the sky. Hold your raised leg with one hand and place your other hand on the hip and thigh of the other leg to feel any shifting in your pelvis.

Holding the pose: Inhale and lengthen your spine on the mat and bring your raised leg further to the sky. Exhale and release your raised leg closer to your body.

Modifications: Bend either leg to ease tension in your hamstrings. If you find that your body lifts off of the mat, use a strap around your raised foot so that you can lower your body to your mat.

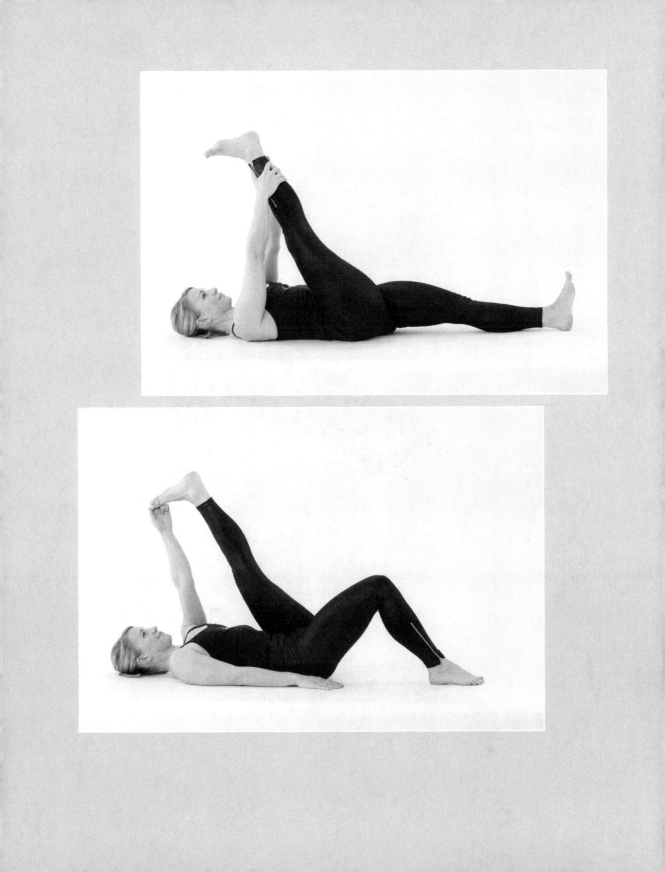

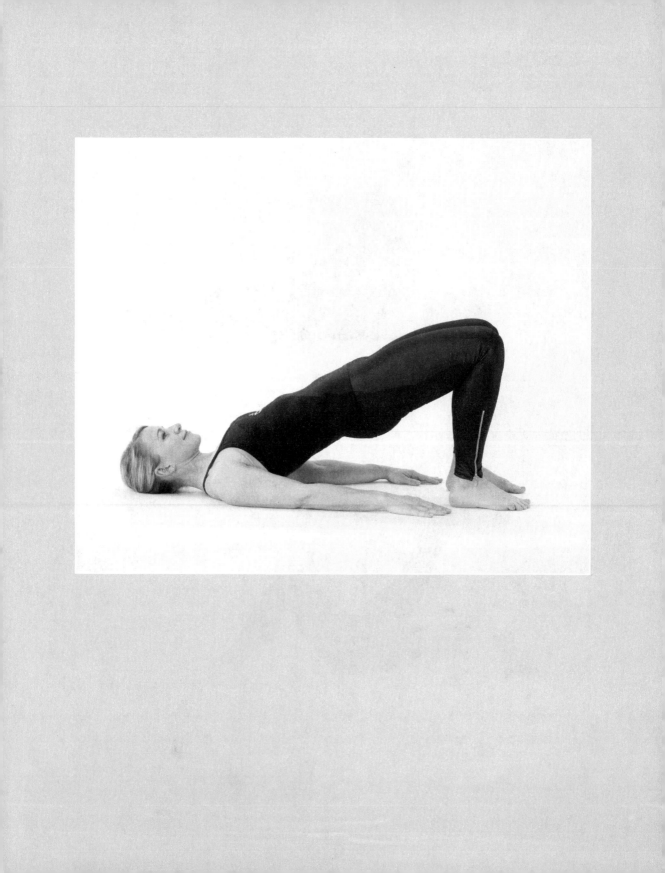

BRIDGE

Benefit of the pose: Bridge strengthens your hamstrings, glutes, and muscles deep in your core center. It relieves tension in the hips from excessive rounding of the spine or long periods of sitting. It offsets the demands of skating and cycling by opening the front of your hips. You can also add a chest expansion here as well.

Getting into the pose: Lie down on your back and bend your knees, placing your feet hip-width apart on your mat. With your arms at your sides, press into your heels and lift your pelvis to the sky.

Holding the pose: Reach your knees away from you and engage your inner thighs. Keep your gaze upward and your head neutral to protect your neck. For the chest expansion option, one at a time, tuck one shoulder underneath you and reach your hands together, interlacing your fingers.

Modifications: Use a block under your hips for a rest in this pose (see page 274). Turn your palms to promote more chest opening and core focus.

Skiing/Snowboarding

When skiing and snowboarding, you spend a lot of your time in a squatting position. Therefore, with yoga poses such as gentle Chair Flow, you will promote proper alignment of the upper and lower body in a squat, and you'll gain an awareness of your movement efficiencies or deficiencies. Because of the quad-dominant activity, it is important to strengthen glutes and hamstrings. These areas are addressed in standing strength poses such as Warrior and Chair.

A common skiing or snowboarding injury is to the wrist—it often takes the brunt of impact and your weight when you fall. A skier's or snowboarder's back also needs attention: The rounded or hunched position while on the slopes is good for aerodynamics but not for posture. You can strengthen both your wrists and your back with yoga poses like Downward Facing Dog. Child's Pose also helps you feel the tuck position, which will help you if you fall.

Both skiing and snowboarding require balance and controlled weight transfer to adapt to varied terrain and steer the course down the hill or mountain. The poses suggested here will provide balance and stability to absorb moguls and jumps, gaining you strength to complete the whole run. Increased body awareness and balance will help you feel your ski edges better, enabling you to execute great turns. Smooth transitions through snowy and icy terrain require a flow of movement associated with overall strength and flexibility. Absorbing moguls, controlled deceleration into corners, and powering up out of turns can all be complemented by Squat (Chair Pose) and the Warrior, Lunge, and Warrior III poses.

Finally, the endurance of holding standing strength poses like Warrior can help you build the stamina to make it down the mountain without breaks, so you can tally up more runs in a day.

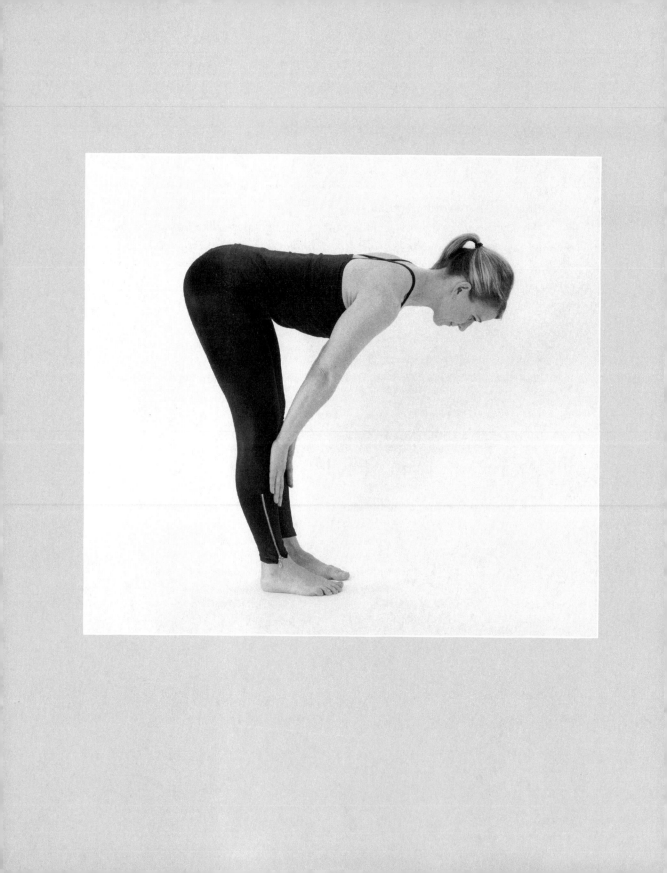

MONKEY

Benefit of the pose: This pose strengthens the entire back, rear shoulder muscles, core center, glutes, and hamstrings. This movement is necessary for safe and effective deadlifts in the weight room. It develops proper form and perhaps an awareness of faulty movement patterns.

Getting into the pose: From Chair, hinge deeper and place your hands on your shins. With a micro bend in your knees, reach your heart forward.

Holding the pose: Continue to reach through the crown of your head and your tailbone to lengthen your spine. Reach your shoulders back and down and imagine a flattened back.

Modifications: Bend your knees more to ease tension through your hamstrings and lower back. For more release, place your hands on your thighs or on a block in front of you for more support while you build strength.

DOWNWARD FACING DOG

(DOWNWARD FACING DOG FLOW)

Benefit of the pose: This pose opens you across your chest and helps you breathe fully through your abdomen. It opens the front of your shoulders while building shoulder strength. It stretches the whole back of your body, including calves, hamstrings, glutes, and major back muscles. This pose releases tension in the body and, through the inversion effect, aids blood flow to your brain. It creates a sense of alertness to prepare you for what comes next. With regular practice this pose can be very restful.

Getting into the pose: From Child's Pose, tuck your toes under and reach your arms ahead. Press into your toes and spread your fingers wide while you lift your hips to the sky. Make an inverted V shape with your body.

Holding the pose: Inhale to reach your tailbone up and lengthen your spine. Exhale to bring your chest and belly toward your thighs.

Modifications: If you have a hard time keeping your spine from rounding, bend your knees to keep your hips hinged and your spine long. To relieve tension in your wrists, come down onto the forearms with your elbows shoulder-width apart. Child's Pose is also an option for a rest at any time.

See also Downward Facing Dog Flow sequence, p. 38.

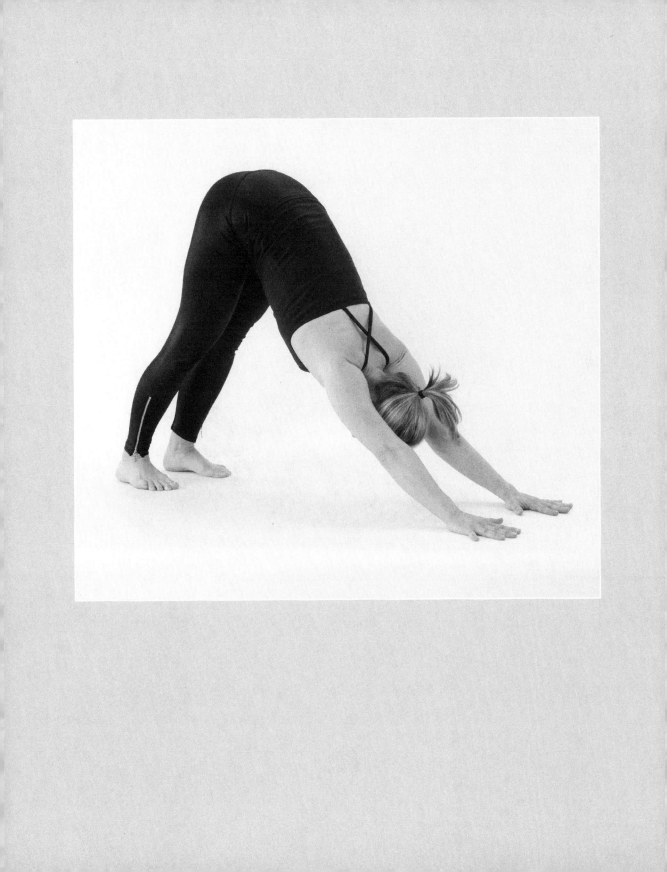

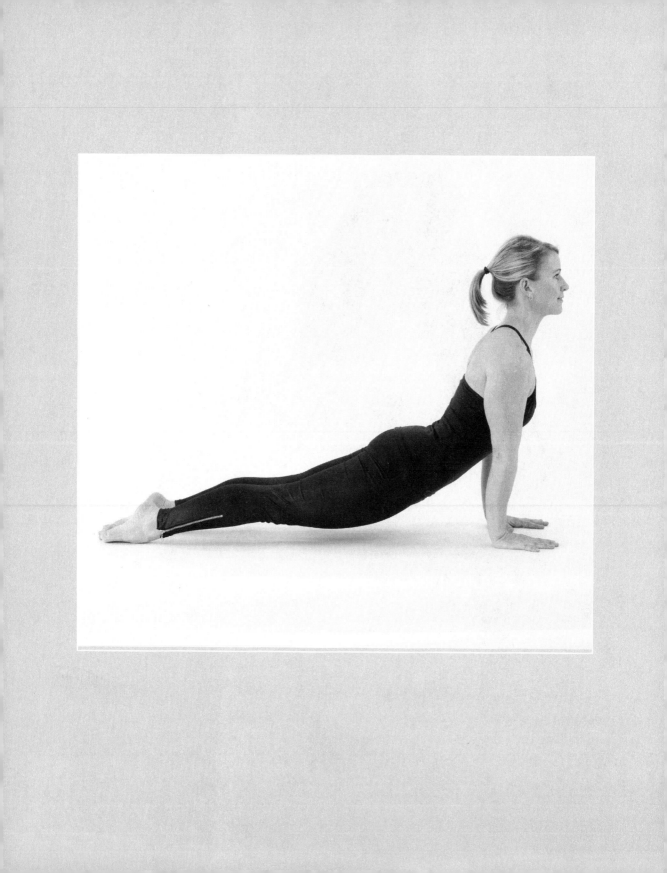

UPWARD FACING DOG or HALF SERIES

Benefit of the pose: Upward Facing Dog strengthens the entire back, lower chest muscles, triceps, and your core center. It also stretches your upper chest and shoulders. Upward Facing Dog is great to use as a flow as in Half Series, see page 40, a more intense option with more work in your shoulders.

Getting into Upward Facing Dog: From Downward Facing Dog, shift forward into Plank and flip your feet so that the tops of your feet are pressing into the mat. Reach through the crown of your head and pull your heart forward. Lower your pelvis but keep your legs off of the mat. Lengthen your arms and reach your shoulders back and down. Engage your pelvic floor and core to protect your lower back.

Holding the pose: Continue to lengthen from head to toe while you lift your navel toward your spine and draw your shoulders back and down. Press away from your mat to support your weight and continue to pull your heart forward.

Modifications: For less intensity, choose Cobra Pose or the Kneeling Half Series, page 42. Feel free to rest back in Child's Pose in case of fatigue.

WARRIOR I

Benefit of the pose: This pose opens up the front of your hips on one side while strengthening your hip and thigh muscles on the other. Upper back muscles are also strengthened by staying lifted through the heart. Warrior poses help to keep our hips mobile and strong.

Getting into the pose: From a standing position, step back with one foot and extend your arms above with your shoulders back and down. Lower your back heel to the floor, keeping your pelvis facing forward.

Holding the pose: Straighten your leg and keep all four corners of your back foot on your mat. Feel the work in the pelvis.

Modifications: If you feel tension in your lower back, lift your heel as in Warrior Lunge or step wider side to side to make room to move your pelvis.

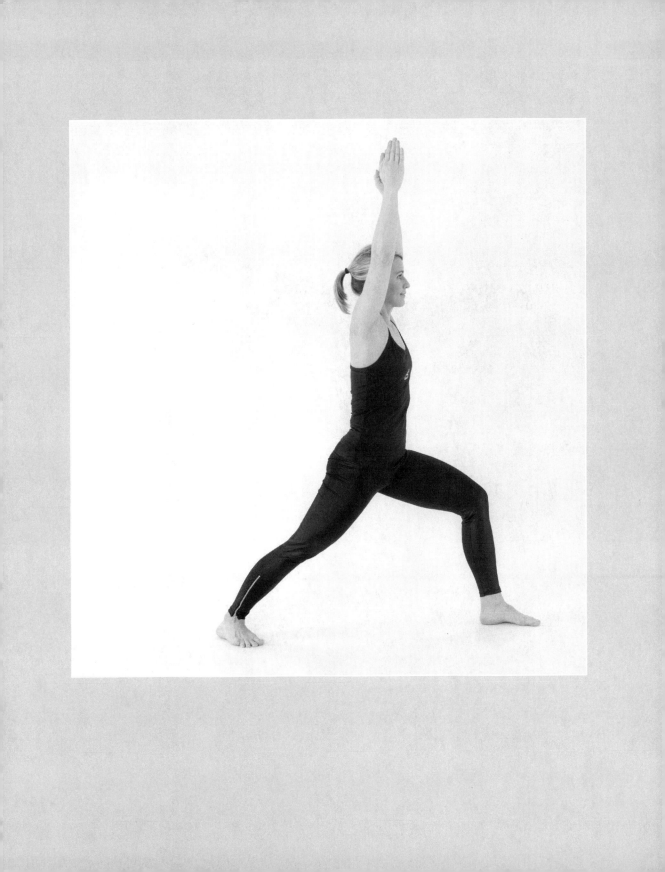

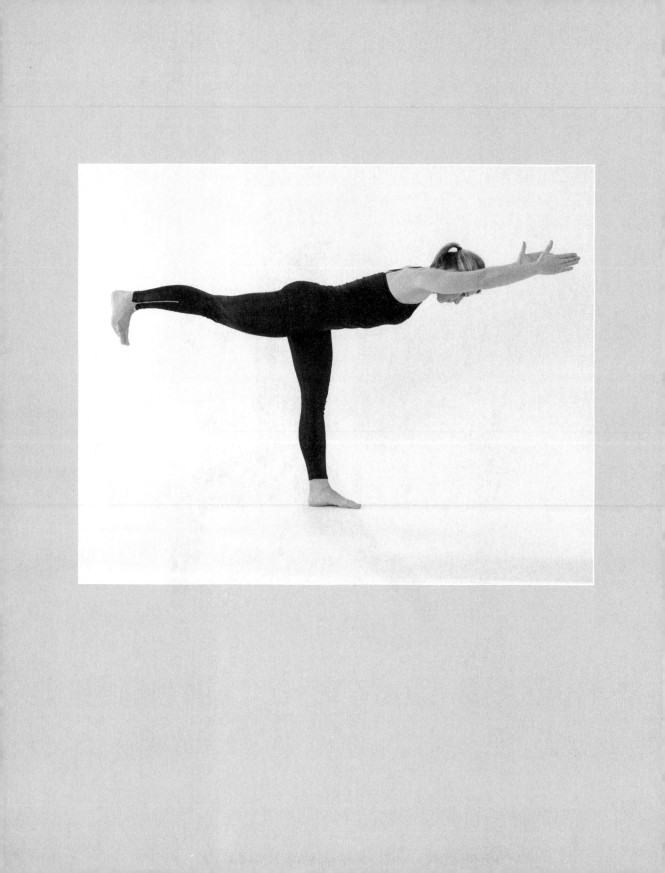

WARRIOR III

Benefit of the pose: Warrior III incorporates strength and balance. It strengthens your hamstrings, glutes, back extensors, hip, and core stabilizers. It also increases focus and concentration. This pose is effective to develop strength and control in movements such as diving and reaching for the ball.

Getting into the pose: From a standing position, extend one leg back and place your hands on your pelvis to start. Keep your pelvis facing forward and hinge forward from the hip of your standing leg and keep a micro bend in the knee. While you dip your upper body down, extend your back leg further up to make a straight line from your heel to the crown of your head and fingertips.

Holding the pose: Reach your arms forward or to the sides and extend the spine to work the core center and strengthen your back muscles. Reach your raised leg away to work the glutes and hamstrings, keeping your hips, knees, and toes pointing to the floor. Stand tall on your supporting leg.

Modifications: For less load on your lower back, bring your arms closer to your body and place your hands together at your heart. To offer support and prevent fatigue, place your hands on your thigh.

THREAD the NEEDLE

Benefit of the pose: This posture stretches your lower back and chest and the rear of one shoulder and the front of the other shoulder. With your head down and your hips up, your spine is not compressed by gravity in this rotation. It reinforces spinal alignment and length across your shoulders through a rotation as well.

Getting into the pose: From all fours, lift one arm forward with your thumb to the sky. Bring your extended arm through the space between your opposite arm and your leg, bringing your shoulder to a resting place on the mat. Engage your core center to support your spine with the rotation. Place your hand on the floor, onto the back of your hip, or extend your arm to the sky to stretch the front of your shoulder and deepen the rotation.

Holding the pose: Your lower shoulder can rest on your mat while you reach up with your other arm. Keep your hips above your knees.

Modifications: Use padding or a folded mat as cushioning for the shoulder or head. Leave your opposite arm on the floor for support to reduce work.

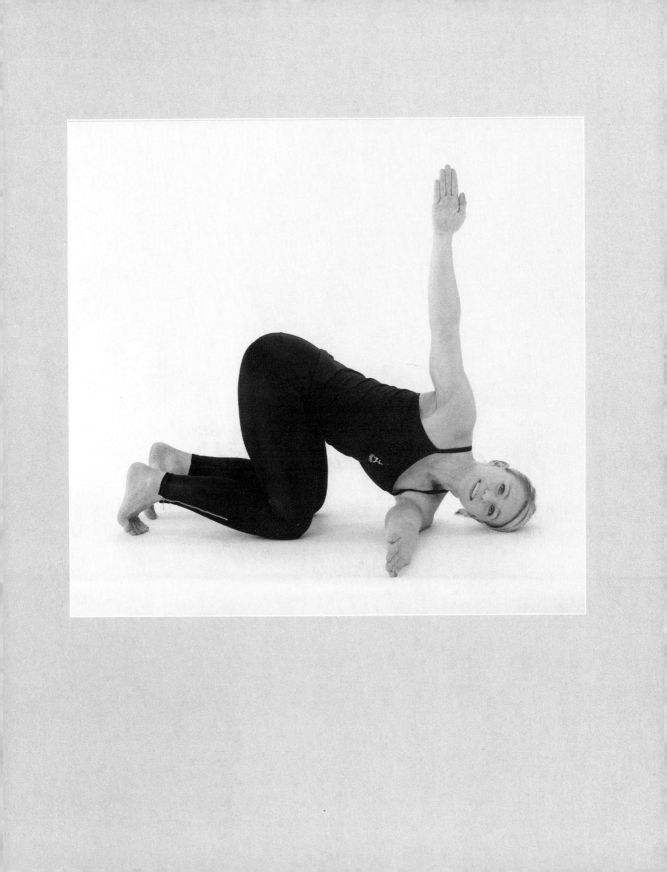

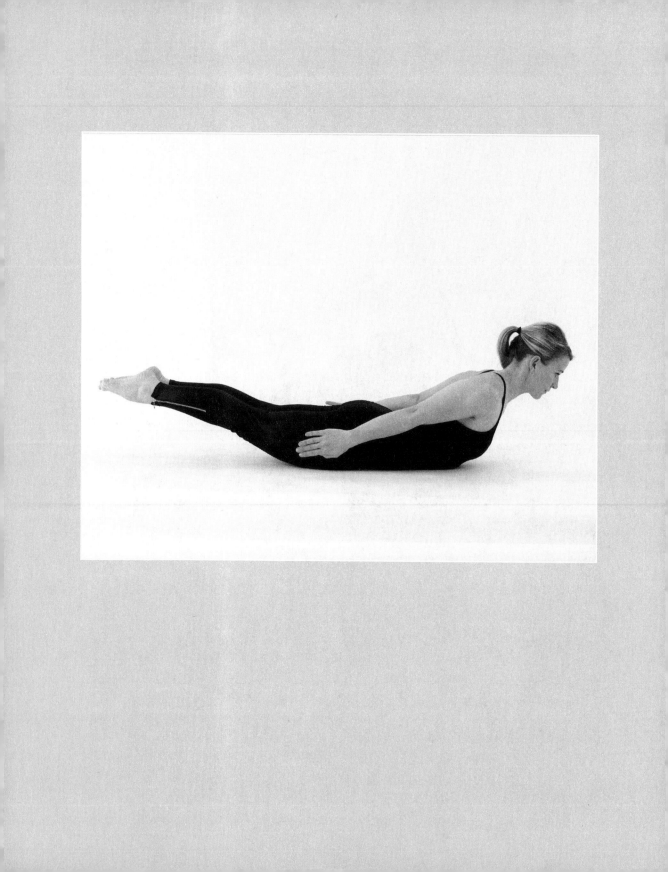

LOCUST

Benefit of the pose: This pose strengthens the entire back of the body, including your hamstrings, glutes, back extensors, upper back, and rear shoulder muscles. It also prepares you for more intense back work in poses like Bow and Camel.

Getting into the pose: From Downward Facing Dog, bring your knees and upper body to the floor. Lie facedown and turn one cheek to the floor with your arms to your sides. Reach with your toes and activate your inner thighs and core center, lifting your belly button to your spine. Reach your shoulder blades toward your spine, lifting your chest and shoulders away from your mat, and let your head follow. Keep your palms facing inward and reach your fingers toward your feet.

Holding the pose: Maintain a good connection through your core center to protect your lower back. Imagine that you are stretched like a hammock and continue to reach your toes and head away, spreading the work throughout your body.

Modifications: For less sensation, bring your hands back to the floor under your shoulders, as in Cobra, for more support. For more sensation, lift your legs away from the floor, keeping your feet together.

Swimming

Swimming is arguably a sport that uses the whole body; strong *side* imbalance is less of an issue but strong muscle group imbalance *is* because you use your body slightly differently depending on your style of swim—freestyle, breaststroke, backstroke, and butterfly. There is not a lot of impact in swimming, so most of the injuries are from repetition or overuse. Because shoulders move through circumduction, full range of motion of your shoulder is important. Developing posture awareness is as important as maintaining strength and mobility through your hips and shoulders. We need to be aware of internal rotation of the shoulder in butterfly, spinal flexion and extension development for breaststroke and butterfly, and knee support for breaststroke.

Swimming requires smooth fluid movement that is wonderfully transferable to a yoga practice. Yoga promotes a strong, agile body, and you can take the controlled yet strength-oriented movements from the mat to the water as well. Energy transfer in the water, regardless of stroke choice, requires full-body movement, a capability of streamlined action in the water, and the ability to propel yourself with your legs. Pulling with strength and consistency is also a skill imperative to a swimmer. Core strength is also key in swimming: The nature of any swimming stroke is an open-chain exercise, meaning that the athlete does not have a solid foundation to push off of or pull toward, thus increasing the requirement for core control to generate movement in the water.

The butterfly stroke in particular exposes an athlete to repeated forceful flexion and extension with the energy transfer to a kick. Strength and length of the back and abdominals can be achieved through Plank, Downward Facing Dog, Locust, and Child's Pose. Swimmers often have tight lateral muscles, but a relaxed yet reaching Child's Pose will help lengthen these powerful pulling muscles.

Lastly, breath control and awareness and the ability to take in deep breaths can enhance and contribute to smooth and fast swimming strokes. We work on breath with every pose.

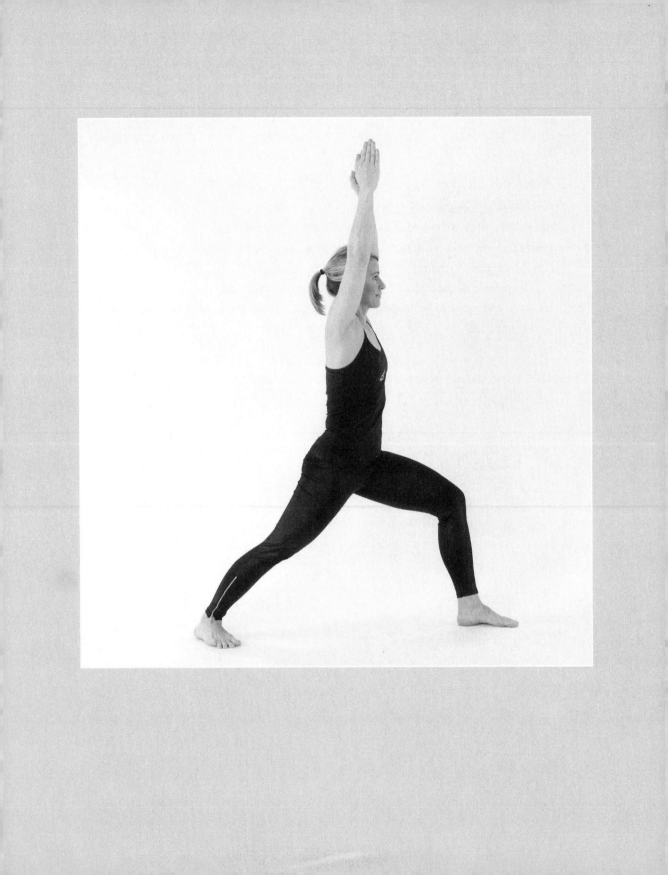

WARRIOR I

Benefit of the pose: This pose opens up the front of your hips on one side while strengthening your hip and thigh muscles on the other. Upper back muscles are also strengthened by staying lifted through the heart. Warrior poses help to keep our hips mobile and strong.

Getting into the pose: From a standing position, step back with one foot and extend your arms above with your shoulders back and down. Lower your back heel to the floor, keeping your pelvis facing forward.

Holding the pose: Straighten your leg and keep all four corners of your back foot on your mat. Feel the work in the pelvis.

Modifications: If you feel tension in your lower back, lift your heel as in Warrior Lunge or step wider side to side to make room to move your pelvis.

WARRIOR II

Benefit of the pose: Warrior II stretches inner thighs and calves while strengthening the quads, glutes, hamstrings, upper back, and shoulders. It increases your ability to deal with stress and improves your focus.

Getting into the pose: From Warrior I/Warrior Lunge, keep your front knee over the ankle. Inhale and lift your body slightly upward and rotate your torso open to the long edge of your mat. Look over your front fingers as you lower your body.

Holding the pose: Reach forward and back with your arms and keep your pelvis directly beneath your ribs. Continue to notice your knee and make sure it stays over the front ankle. Engage your core center and lift through the top of your head to stay long through your torso. Relax your shoulders back and down.

Modifications: For less intensity, shorten your stance and be up a little higher. To relieve tension in the neck and shoulders, bring your hands to your heart.

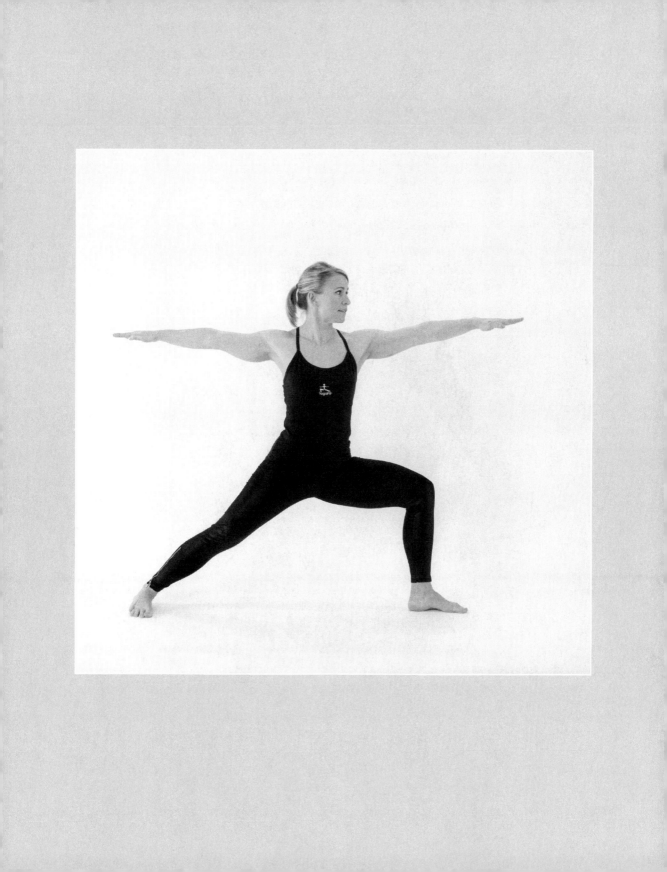

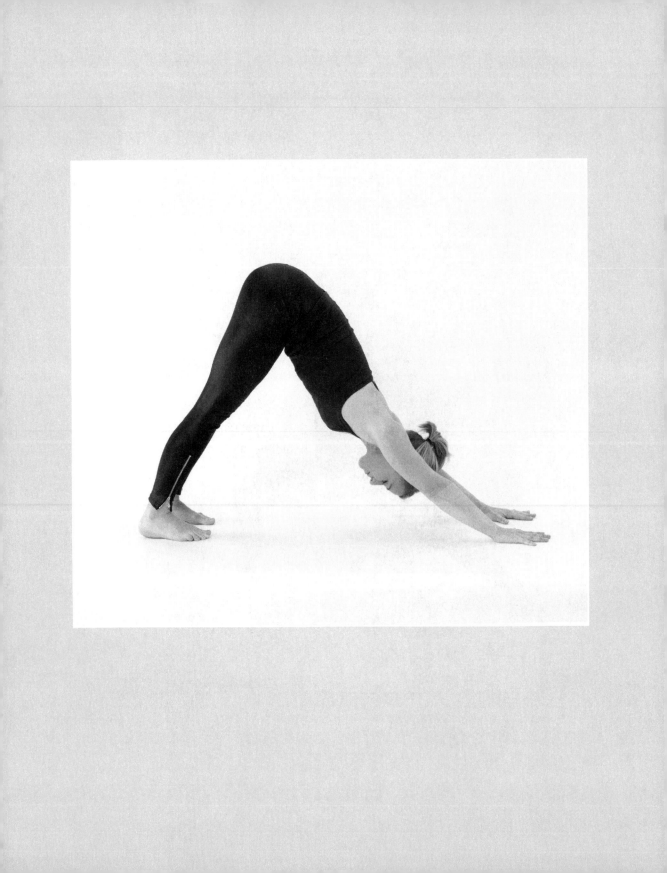

DOWNWARD FACING DOG

Benefit of the pose: This pose opens you across your chest and helps you breathe fully through your abdomen. It opens the front of your shoulders while building shoulder strength. It stretches the whole back of your body, including calves, hamstrings, glutes, and major back muscles. This pose releases tension in the body and, through the inversion effect, aids blood flow to your brain. It creates a sense of alertness to prepare you for what comes next. With regular practice this pose can also be very restful.

Getting into the pose: From Child's Pose, tuck your toes under and reach your arms ahead. Press into your toes and spread your fingers wide while you lift your hips to the sky. Make an inverted V shape with your body.

Holding the pose: Inhale to reach your tailbone up and lengthen your spine. Exhale to bring your chest and belly toward your thighs.

Modifications: If you have a hard time keeping your spine from rounding, bend your knees to keep your hips hinged and your spine long. To relieve tension in your wrists, come down onto the forearms with your elbows shoulder-width apart. Child's Pose is also an option for a rest at any time.

SPINAL BALANCE

Benefit of the pose: Spinal Balance encourages your core center muscles to stabilize as you resist gravity. It also strengthens your glutes, upper and lower back, chest, and shoulders.

Getting into the pose: From your hands and knees, stabilize your shoulders and hips. Extend one arm out at the height of your shoulder. Lift the opposite leg just to the height of your hips.

Holding the pose: Keep a long line from your fingers to your heel and hold for 5–10 breaths. Focus on stability and strength while you lift your navel to your spine. You may also flow this pose: Inhale as you lengthen your arm and leg and exhale as you bring them back to the floor, then switch sides. Continue to reach forward with your fingers and press back through your heel, toes to the floor, with little or no movement in the torso. Repeat 5–10 times per side.

Modifications: To relieve wrist tension, use fists for wrists, palms facing each other. For knee comfort, place padding or make a fold in the mat to kneel on. For less sensation, extend just the arm or just the leg.

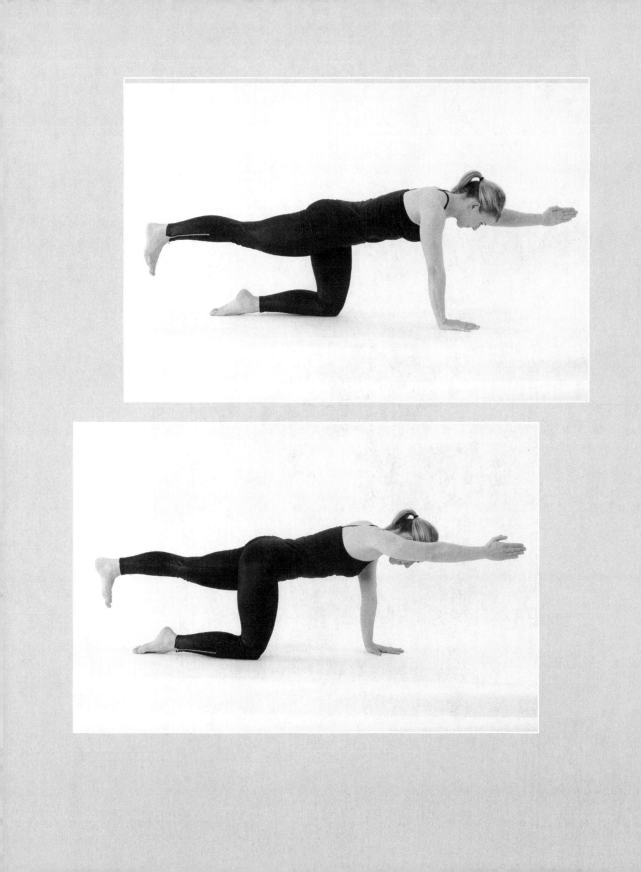

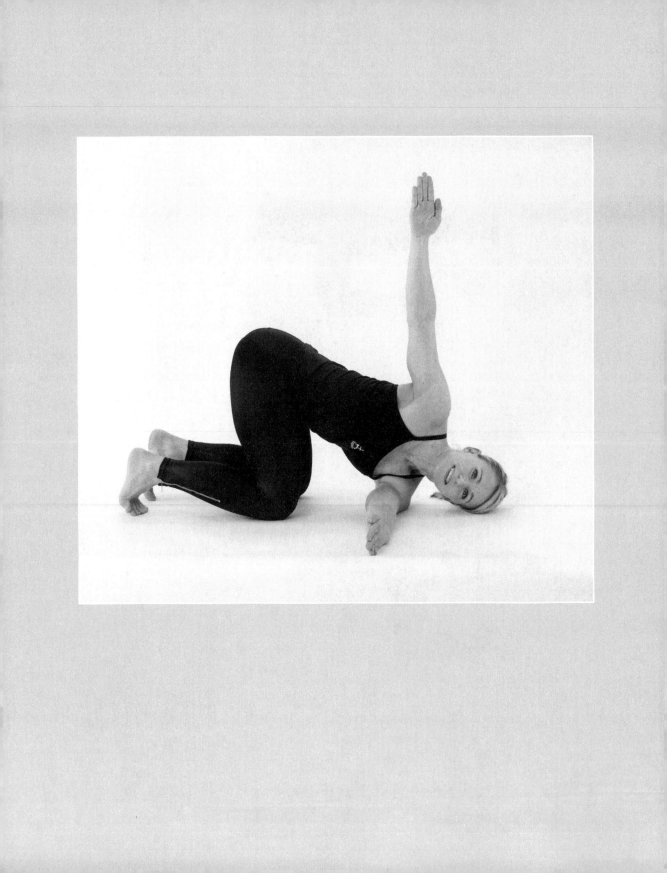

THREAD the NEEDLE

Benefit of the pose: This posture stretches your lower back and chest and the rear of one shoulder and the front of the other shoulder. With your head down and your hips up, your spine is not compressed by gravity in this rotation. It reinforces spinal alignment and length across your shoulders through a rotation as well.

Getting into the pose: From all fours, lift one arm forward with your thumbs to the sky. Bring your extended arm through the space between your opposite arm and your leg, bringing your shoulder to a resting place on the mat. Engage your core center to support your spine with the rotation. Place the opposite hand on the floor, onto the back of your hip, or extend your arm to the sky to stretch the front of your shoulder and deepen the rotation.

Holding the pose: Your lower shoulder can rest on your mat while you reach up with your other arm. Keep your hips above your knees.

Modifications: Use padding or a folded mat as cushioning for the shoulder or head. Leave your opposite arm on the floor for support to reduce work.

PLANK (WITH SINGLE LEG LIFT/EXTENSION)

Benefit of the pose: This pose strengthens your entire body. Using good posture techniques as you would when standing, you are now holding your weight above the ground. It strengthens the shoulders, chest, lower back, core, glutes, hamstrings, quads, and even muscles in the hands, wrists, feet, and ankles. With the leg extension, you intensify the work in your core center and upper body, and it targets the glute and hamstring of your raised leg. Holding the leg lift can strengthen a swimmer's kick.

Getting into the pose: From Downward Facing Dog, shift forward so that your shoulders are directly above your wrists. Lengthen your legs and position your pelvis to create a smooth, straight line from your ankles to the crown of your head. With a flexed foot, lift one leg from the hip and keep your pelvis level and your spine long.

Holding the pose: Lift your belly button to your spine and reach through the crown of your head. Use breath and dynamic tension to spread the work through the entire body.

Modifications: If your lower back drops or your shoulders are up around your ears, choose Kneeling Plank. This will ease tension and reduce the workload while you develop upper body strength.

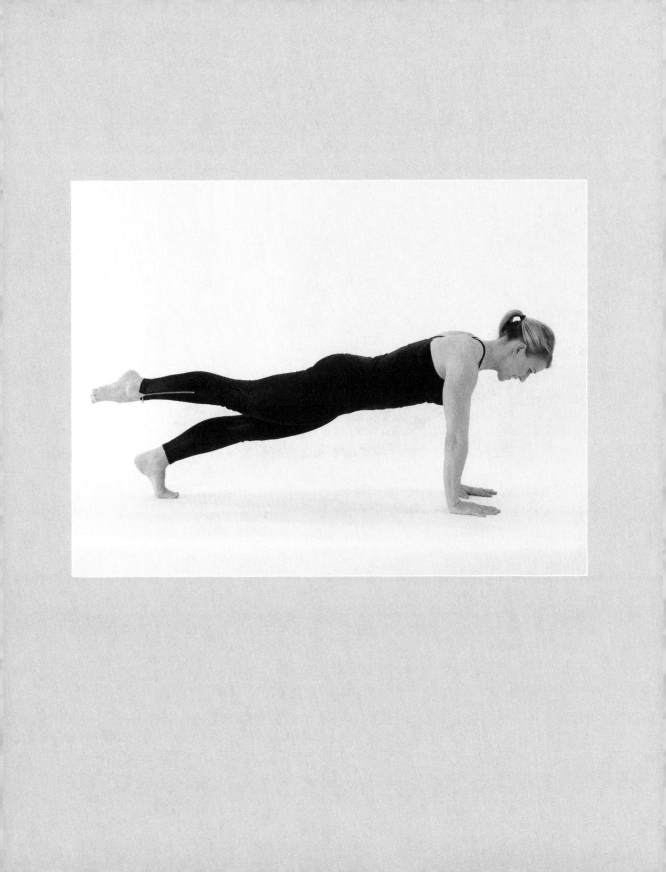

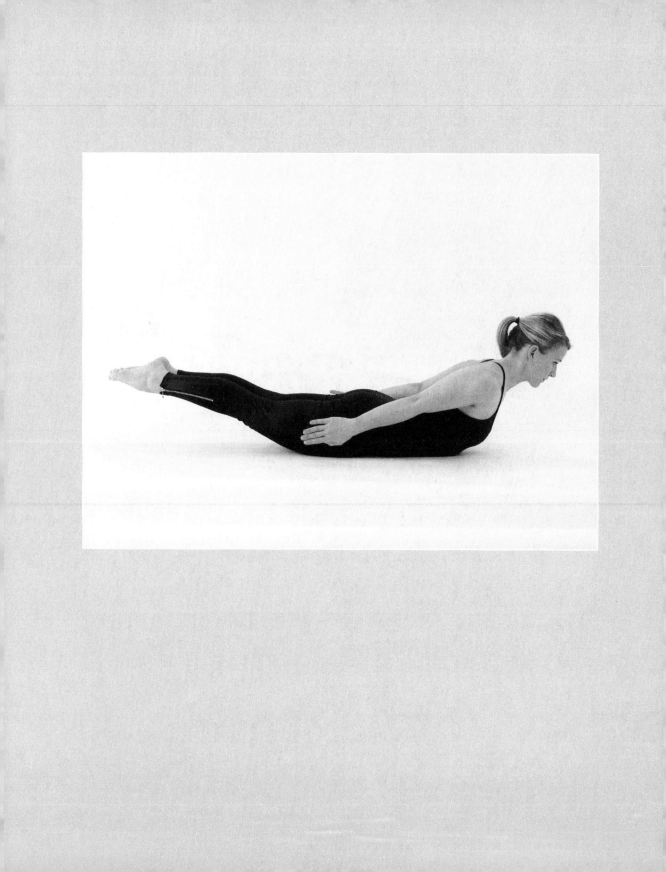

LOCUST

Benefit of the pose: This pose strengthens the entire back of the body, including your hamstrings, glutes, back extensors, upper back, and rear shoulder muscles. It also prepares you for more intense back work in poses like Bow and Camel.

Getting into the pose: Lie facedown and turn one cheek to the floor with your arms to your sides. Reach with your toes and activate your inner thighs and core center*, lifting your belly away from the floor. Reach your shoulder blades toward your spine, lifting your chest and shoulders away from your mat, and let your head follow. Keep your palms facing inward and reach your fingers toward your feet.

Holding the pose: Maintain a good connection through your core center* to protect your lower back. Imagine that you are stretched like a hammock and continue to reach your toes and head away, spreading the work throughout your body.

Modifications: For less sensation, bring your hands back to the floor under your shoulders, as in Cobra, for more support. For more sensation, lift your legs away from the floor, keeping your feet together.

CHILD'S POSE

Benefit of the pose: Child's Pose is often used to offset the intensity of intense back extensions, a counter pose. Child's Pose is grounding, relaxing, and soothing to the body physically and energetically. When sports activity demands high levels of intensity, alertness, action, and reaction, levels of cortisol (a stress hormone) rise. Child's Pose is very restorative.

Getting into the pose: From your belly, press back to bring your hips toward your heels. From a kneeling position, reach your hands out in front on the floor and lower your body to your thighs.

Holding the pose: Your arms can stay over your head or you can put them along your sides. Use your breath and gravity to relax and let go. With your arms overhead, you can easily make transitions into other poses.

Modifications: Widen your knees to clear space for your belly. If your hips or knees are uncomfortable, place some padding under or behind your knees. You may also leave your hips up higher to relieve tension.

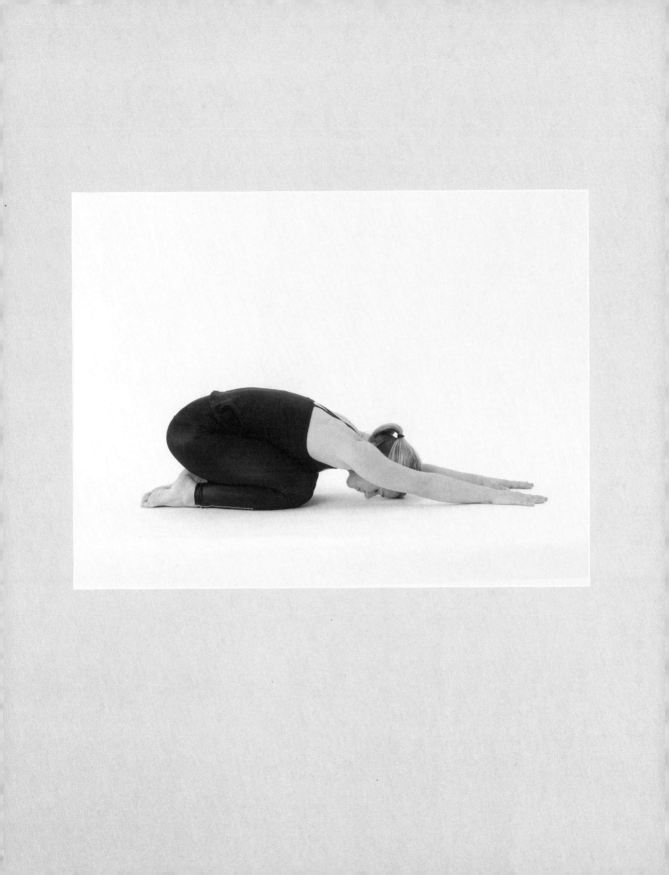

cool-down: final stretch and flex sequence

No matter what your chosen activity is, it is just as important to incorporate a cool-down as it is to incorporate a warmup. It is necessary for the body to gradually return to its normal temperature, heart rate, and blood flow rate. In addition, this is the time to use static (hold) stretches to help increase your joint range of motion and address commonly tight areas. Expect improved flexibility and mobility with the regular practice of these cool-down poses:

COOL-DOWN POSES

Downward Facing Dog—p. 229

Pigeon—p. 230

Butterfly—p. 233

Bridge—p. 234

Supine Spinal Twist—p. 237

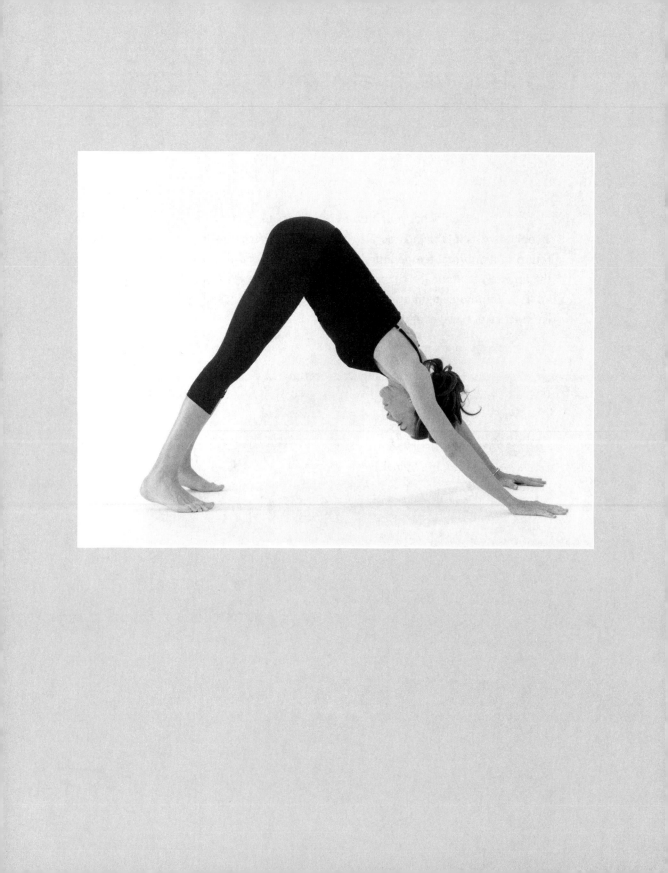

DOWNWARD FACING DOG

Benefit of the pose: This pose opens you across your chest and helps you breathe fully through your abdomen. It opens the front of your shoulders while building shoulder strength. It stretches the whole back of your body, including calves, hamstrings, glutes, and major back muscles. This pose releases tension in the body and, through the inversion effect, aids blood flow to your brain. It creates a sense of alertness to prepare you for what comes next. With regular practice this pose can also be very restful.

Getting into the pose: From Child's Pose, tuck your toes under and reach your arms ahead. Press into your toes and spread your fingers wide while you lift your hips to the sky. Make an inverted V shape with your body.

Holding the pose: Inhale to reach your tailbone up and lengthen your spine. Exhale to bring your chest and belly toward your thighs.

Modifications: If you have a hard time keeping your spine from rounding, bend your knees to keep your hips hinged and your spine long. To relieve tension in your wrists, come down onto the forearms with your elbows shoulder-width apart. Child's Pose is also an option for a rest at any time.

PIGEON

Benefit of the pose: Great for releasing tension and stress, Pigeon stretches the deep glute muscles in the back of the hips. It also helps to stretch the band of muscle that runs down the outside of the thigh from the hip to the knee that gets tight with a lot of running (IT Band).

Getting into the pose: From Downward Facing Dog, bring one leg forward to the floor with your knee bent and your foot flexed. Stay lifted enough to keep your pelvis level.

Holding the pose: Release your upper body down to the floor and rest your forehead on your stacked fists.

Modifications: To make this pose more restorative, lie on your back with your knees bent and your feet on the floor. Lift one leg and place your foot on your other thigh for support. Reach to hold the supporting leg behind the knee and draw your leg in toward your chest. If your range of motion allows, Standing Pigeon from Chair Pose is another option. Bring one ankle to the top of the opposite thigh with your foot flexed and sit back into Chair Pose.

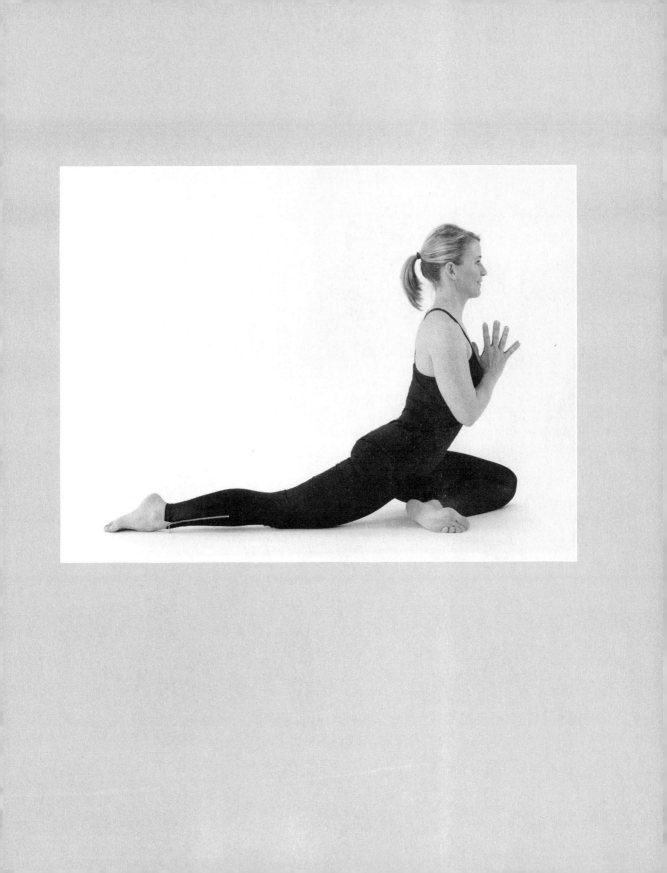

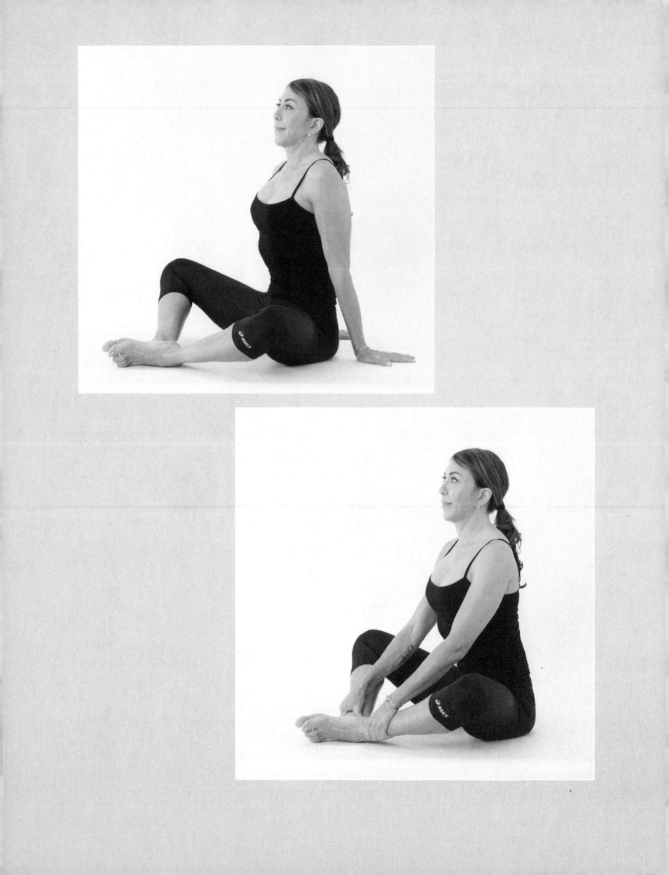

BUTTERFLY

Benefit of the pose: This pose is another great hip opener and very accessible from a seated position. It stretches your hip adductors, glutes, and lower back, releasing tension in your hips and thighs.

Getting into the pose: From Downward Facing Dog, lower your knees to the floor and lower your hips to one side. Swing your legs around and sit tall and place the soles of your feet together about one foot's distance from your groin. Lift through the crown of your head and bring your belly forward.

Holding the pose: Keep your arms along the sides of your rib cage. Keep your elbows pointing back so that you don't push on your legs with them. For more sensation, engage the glutes to draw your knees to the mat.

Modifications: If you feel tight or restricted in movement, sit on a block or a rolled mat. This will also help reduce any rounding in the lower back. Another option is to place your hands on the floor behind you and reach your belly forward with your chest up.

BRIDGE

Benefit of the pose: Bridge strengthens your hamstrings, glutes, and muscles deep in your core center. It relieves tension in the hips from excessive rounding of the spine or long periods of sitting. It offsets the demands of skating and cycling by opening the front of your hips. You can also add a chest expansion here as well.

Getting into the pose: Lie down on your back and bend your knees, placing your feet hip-width apart on your mat. With your arms at your sides, press into your heels and lift your pelvis to the sky.

Holding the pose: Reach your knees away from you and engage your inner thighs. Keep your gaze upward and your head neutral to protect your neck. For the chest expansion option, one at a time, tuck one shoulder underneath you and reach your hands together, interlacing your fingers.

Modifications: Use a block under your hips for a rest in this pose (see page 274). Turn your palms to promote more chest opening and core focus.

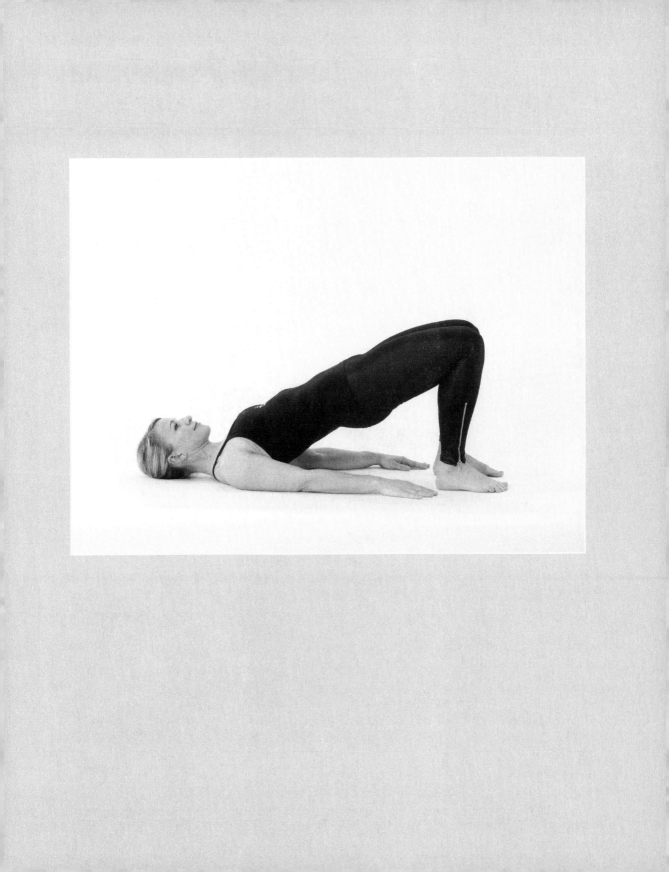

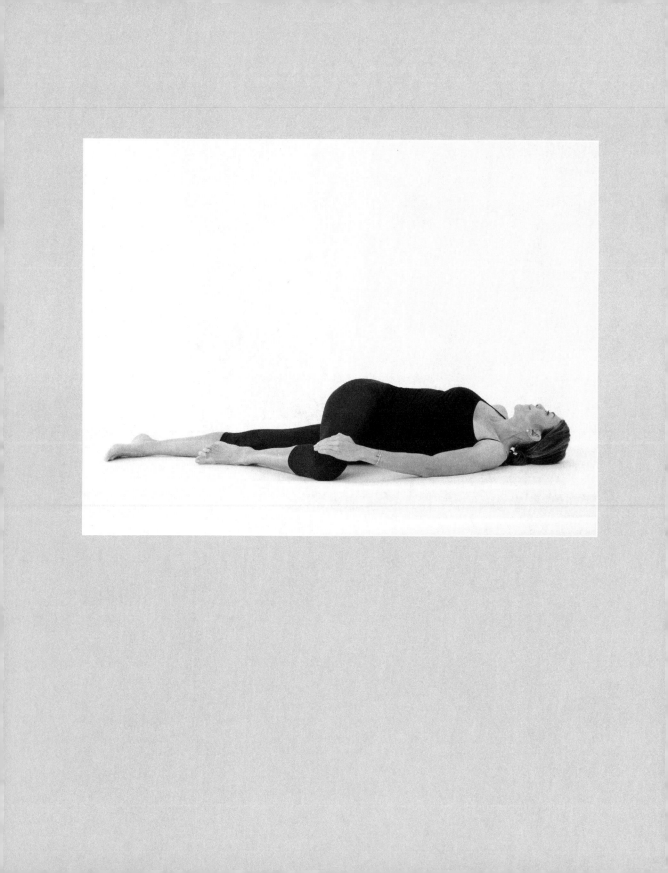

SUPINE SPINAL TWIST

Benefit of the pose: This pose will help you stretch out your lower back and open up your thoracic spine. From a lying position you can lengthen your spine with ease because you don't need to work against gravity. The twist invigorates your torso muscles, stimulates conductivity of your sensory nerves, and massages your internal organs.

Getting into the pose: Lie on the mat on your back and bring your right knee to a bent position with your foot on the floor beside your left leg. Press into your foot and lift your pelvis up enough to shift your pelvis to the right and then rest it on the floor. Keep your right shoulder on the mat and use your left hand to gently draw your right knee over your left and toward the floor.

Holding the pose: Keep both shoulders placed on the mat and look over your left shoulder to maximize the benefit of the twist. Practice releasing toward the floor with every exhale, then switch sides.

Modifications: From a side-lying position, rotate your upper body open, keeping your hips facing the side. Place a block or two under your right knee or a rolled-up mat lengthwise behind you for support. If you have any disc injuries, this pose may aggravate the injury. In this case, start with both knees bent and allow both legs to go to one side.

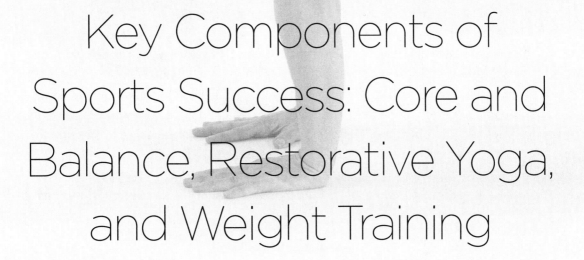

3.

Key Components of Sports Success: Core and Balance, Restorative Yoga, and Weight Training

core and balance poses

No matter your sport of focus, it is crucial to train your core and hone your balance because, as you've already learned, the core is the epicenter of your total body strength, and balance is the root of much of your movement. Many people think of their core as the midsection only, but engaging the core is actually a lot more than your "six-pack." Your core muscles begin at the top of your abdominal trunk and run down to your lower torso, and touch upon all areas of your body with the exception of your arms and legs. There are close to thirty—yes, thirty—muscles attached to the core, all of which we will address in the following workout.

Whether you are running, lifting, or performing activities for the upper and lower body, power in every move comes from the core. Broadening your awareness of it and devoting specific training to its strength will support your overall movement and functionality. This section offers you a number of the poses you've encountered within the sport-specific coverage; use these poses anytime and to complement any sport-specific training. If you are suffering from or have a history of knee ailments, please avoid this exercise.

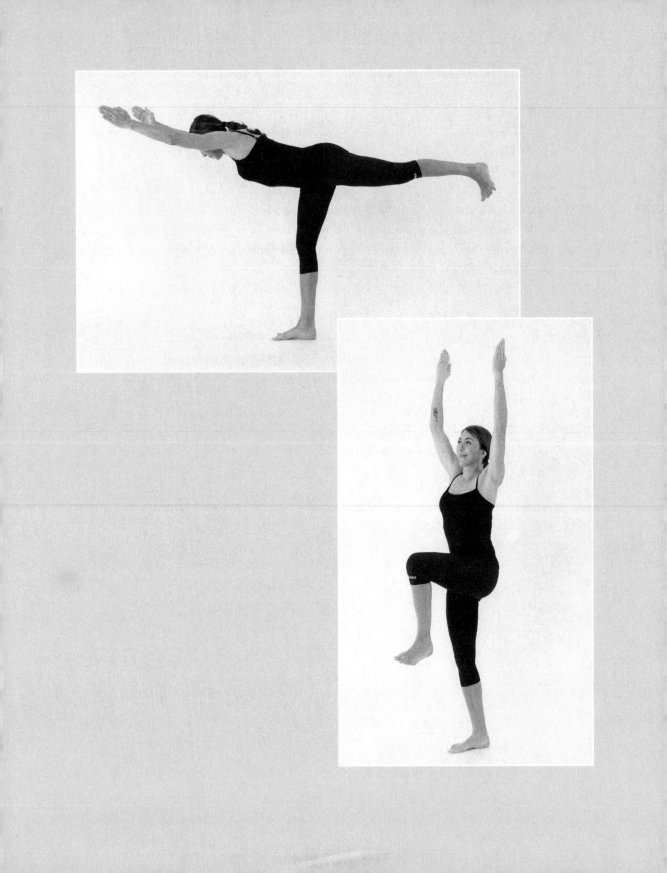

WARRIOR III to LEG UP

Benefit of the pose: Warrior III strengthens your core center, glutes, hamstrings, and entire back. It also improves hip stability and strength within the complex hip joint and develops good technique for single-leg deadlifts. Leg Up stretches your hamstrings and glutes and strengthens your quads.

Getting into Warrior III: From a standing position, shift your weight over to your right foot and keep your pelvis facing forward. Extend your left leg back so that your toes are touching the mat behind you and keep your hips stable. With your hands at your hips to start, hinge forward on your right leg while you lift your left leg up, keeping your spine long and your raised leg straight.

Holding Warrior III: Keep your pelvis facing the floor as well as the knee and toe of your raised leg. Press back through your heel and reach forward through the crown of your head. For more core work, extend your arms ahead of you with your shoulders down and back.

Transition to Leg Up: From Warrior III, lift your upper body back to standing while you lower the extended leg and bring it through to a raised position in front of you with a 90-degree bend at your hip and knee.

Holding Leg Up: Continue to reach your arms up to encourage good posture with core center activation. For a challenge, move with breath from one pose to the other. Inhale to Leg Up and exhale to Warrior III. Repeat 5–10 times.

Modifications: If there is tension in your lower back in Warrior III, bring your arms to your sides or reach behind you. You can also place your hands on your front thigh for support and to prevent fatigue. If you are feeling a little wobbly in Leg Up, then start off with one hand touching the wall.

STANDING PIGEON to TREE POSE

Benefit of the pose: Pigeon stretches the outside of your thighs and the back of your hips. In a standing position, it strengthens your quads with a single-leg squat while you improve your balance. Tree strengthens your hamstrings and glutes and improves your balance and overall posture.

Getting into Standing Pigeon: From Mountain Pose, shift your weight to your right leg and lift your left. Flex your left foot and cross it over to rest your left ankle on your right thigh while you sit back, as in Chair Pose.

Holding the pose: Enjoy the hold for 3–5 breaths while you sit deeper into the stretch.

Getting into Tree: From Standing Pigeon, stand tall on your right leg, move your left foot to the inside of your right leg below or above your knee.

Holding the pose: Hold for 3–5 breaths while you extend your arms like branches or reach up over your head. Switch sides.

Modifications: For ease in holding your foot up on your leg in Pigeon, you may use a strap. For support while your balance improves, you may lean on a wall or a chair.

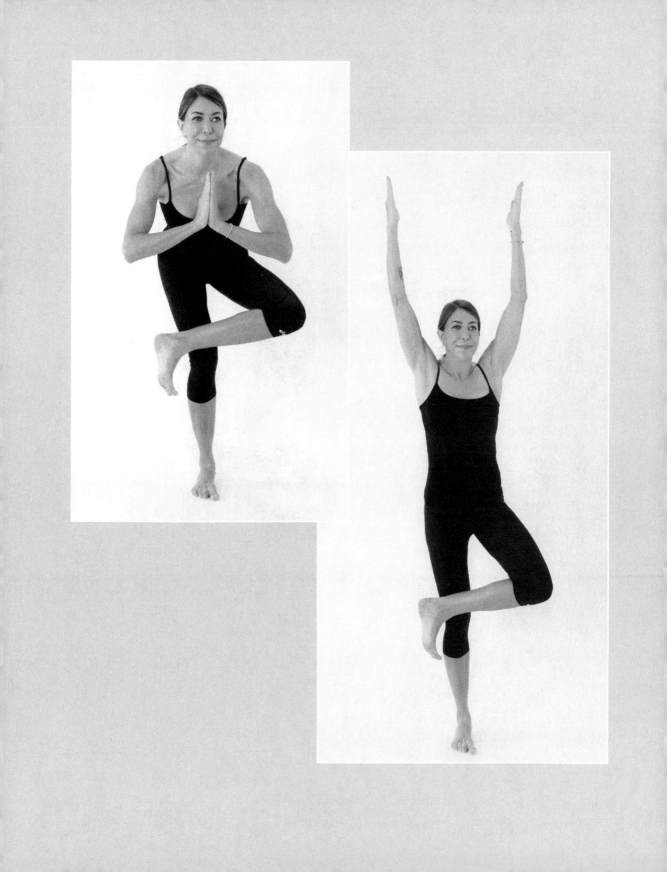

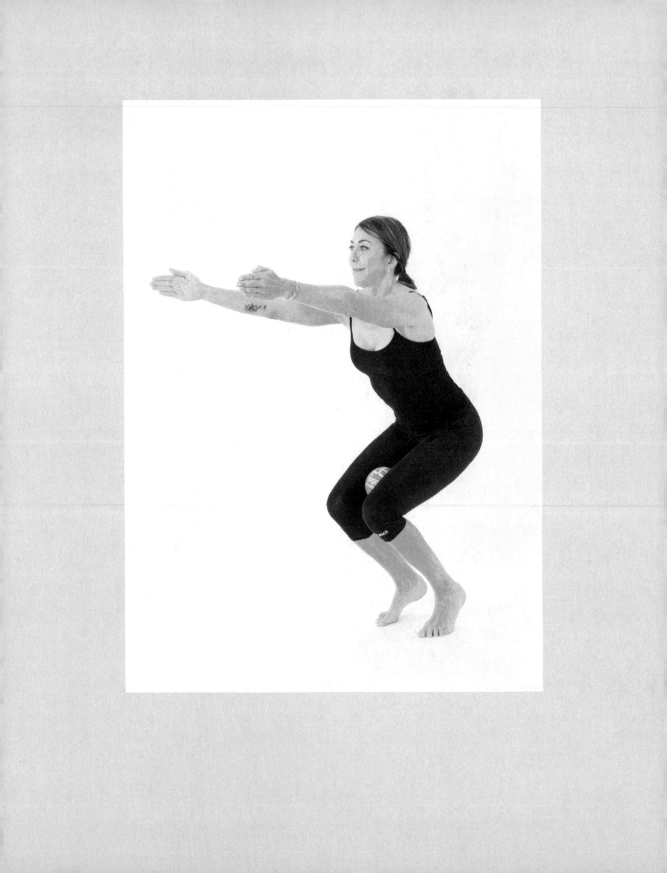

BALANCING CHAIR with CORE BALL

Benefit of the pose: Chair strengthens your quads, glutes, and your entire back. Balancing Chair requires more work for your quads and calves. With the core ball, you work your inner thigh and core center. This pose helps develop good squat technique with heightened awareness to your core center and upper back extension.

Getting into the pose: Place the core ball between your thighs a little above your knees and squeeze the ball just enough to hold it there. Hinge your hips back into Chair Pose, keeping your core center strong and your chest open. Hold your squat position and lift your heels one at a time into Balancing Chair. Keep your shoulders back and down and lift your chest more to keep your weight centered over your raised heels.

Holding the pose: Stay in a seated position and reach your hips back and lift your heart, extending your upper back while holding this pose. Inhale to lengthen your spine and exhale to find more stability.

Modifications: Lower your heels when necessary. If there is tension in the lower back, bring your arms closer to your body, even rest them on your thighs. This will also help reduce tension in your neck and shoulders. To enhance Chair Pose further, you can continue to hold the ball steady and move into Revolving Chair with the ball.

FOCUS on the BALL

Benefit of the pose: This pose is essentially an enhanced Warrior III pose that uses a focal point while you improve balance and strength in your core center.

Getting into the pose: From Mountain, shift your weight over to your right foot and keep your pelvis facing forward. Extend your left leg back so that your toes are touching the mat behind you and keep your hips stable and your leg straight. Reach the ball ahead of you while you hinge forward on your right leg and lift your left leg up, keeping your spine long and your raised leg straight.

Holding the pose: Keep your focus on the ball while you maintain a lengthened torso. Press back through your heel and reach forward with the ball.

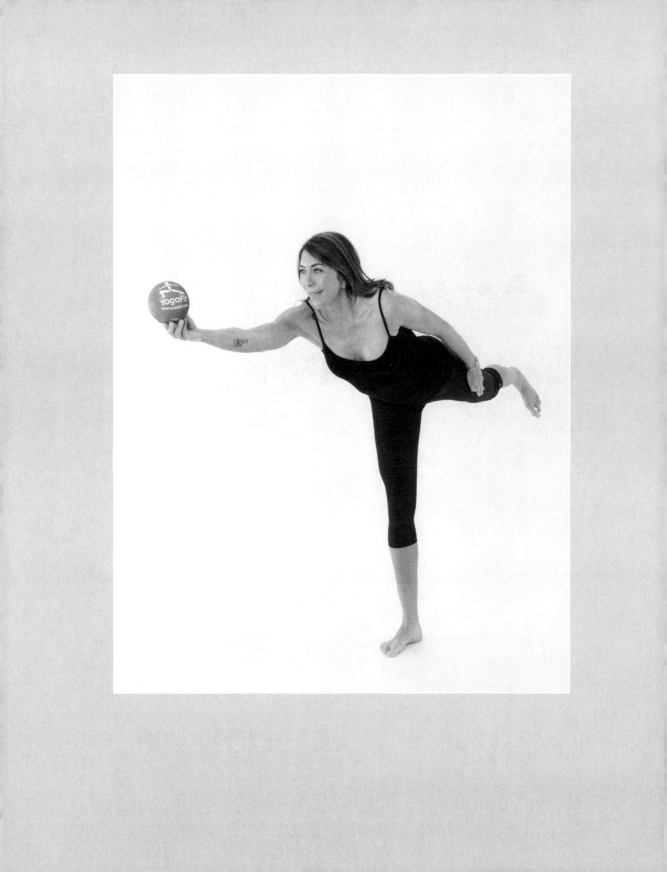

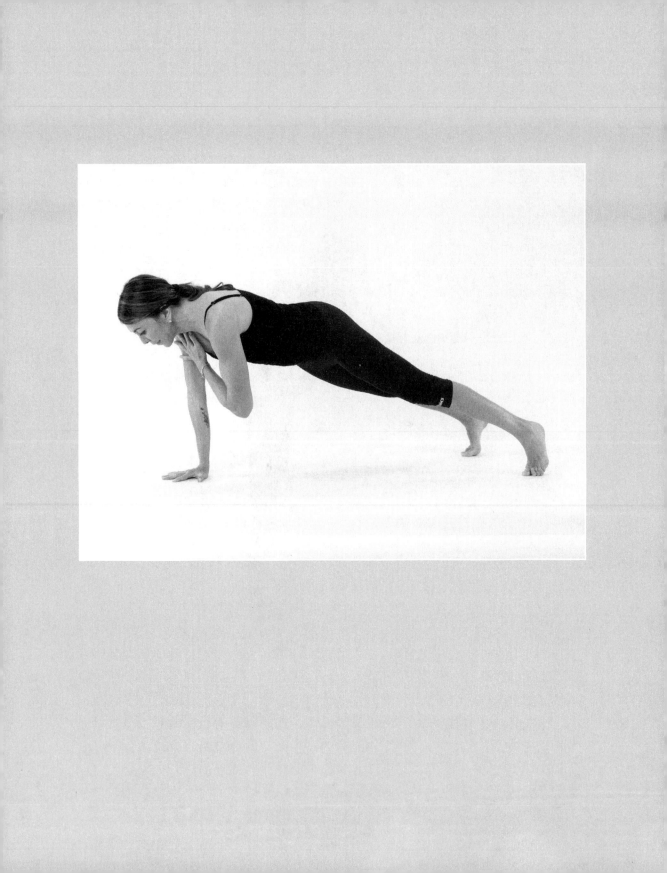

SHOULDER TOUCHES in PLANK POSE
(20–30 REPS)

Benefit of the pose: This works many stabilizers in the core center and shoulder girdle.

Getting into the pose: With your toes on the floor, shift forward so that your shoulders are directly over your wrists. Stabilize your shoulders against your rib cage without squeezing them together. Reach long from your heels to the crown of your head with a strong core center. Lift one hand to touch the opposite shoulder with little or no movement in your torso. Hold and switch sides. Move slowly and steadily to increase awareness of your entire body from your heels to the crown of your head with special attention to your core center and shoulder stability.

Modifications: Move your feet apart for more stability or lower your knees to your mat for a less intense option.

KNEE to SAME ELBOW in PLANK

From Downward Facing Dog, reach one leg back and up. Slowly bring your leg underneath you with a bent knee. Lift up with your core center and reach your knee to your elbow on the same side.

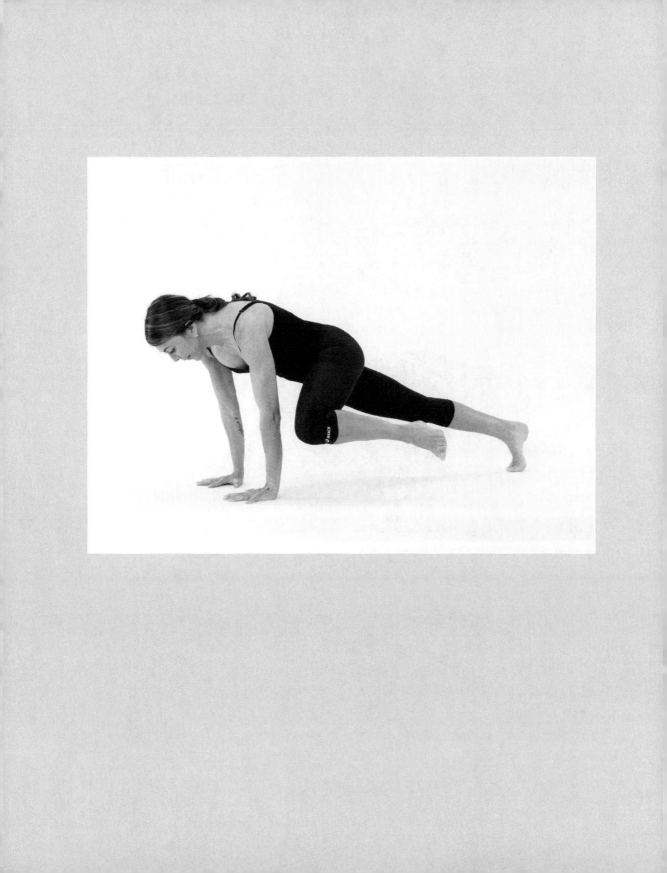

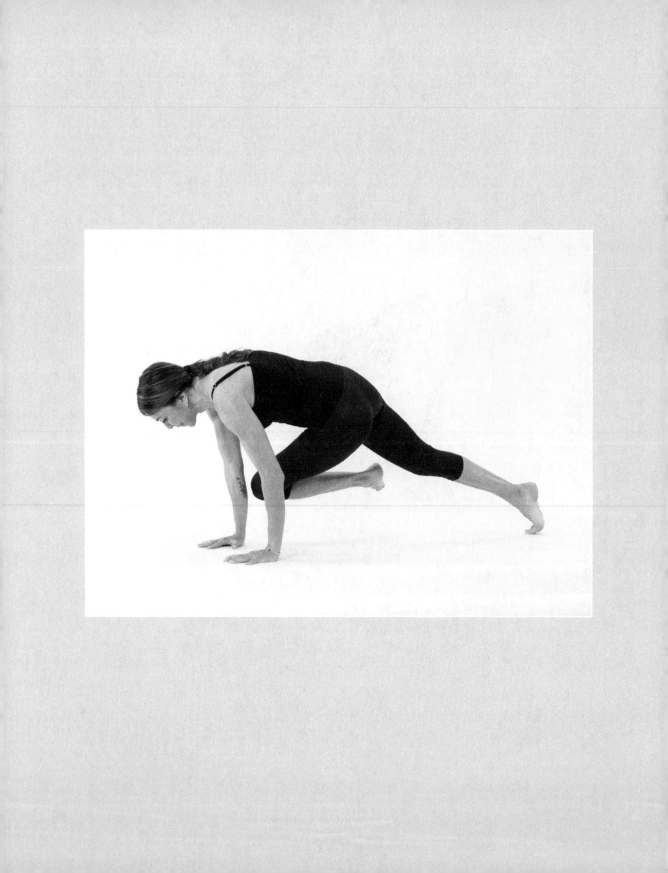

KNEE to OPPOSITE ELBOW in PLANK

From Downward Facing Dog, reach one leg back and up. Slowly bring your leg underneath you with a bent knee. Lift up with your core center and reach your knee to your opposite elbow.

Repeat 1 and 2 (15 reps per side)

Modifications: In one repetition, you may bring your bent knee to your elbow on the same side, then rotate your torso and reach your knee to your opposite elbow, then extend your leg back.

OPENING CLOSING SIDE PLANK POSE

Benefit of the pose: This exercise strengthens your upper body and works to stabilize your shoulders and your core center. Through the rotation, it also strengthens your obliques.

Getting into the pose: From Plank, stabilize your shoulders, making sure that they are directly over your wrists. Lift one arm up and open into Side Plank. Use your oblique muscles to lift your hip to the sky while you reach further with your arm. Take your raised arm and reach it down and under you while you stay lifted in your hips. Lift your arm back up and repeat.

Modifications: If this exercise is too intense on the shoulders, Kneeling Side Plank will decrease intensity.

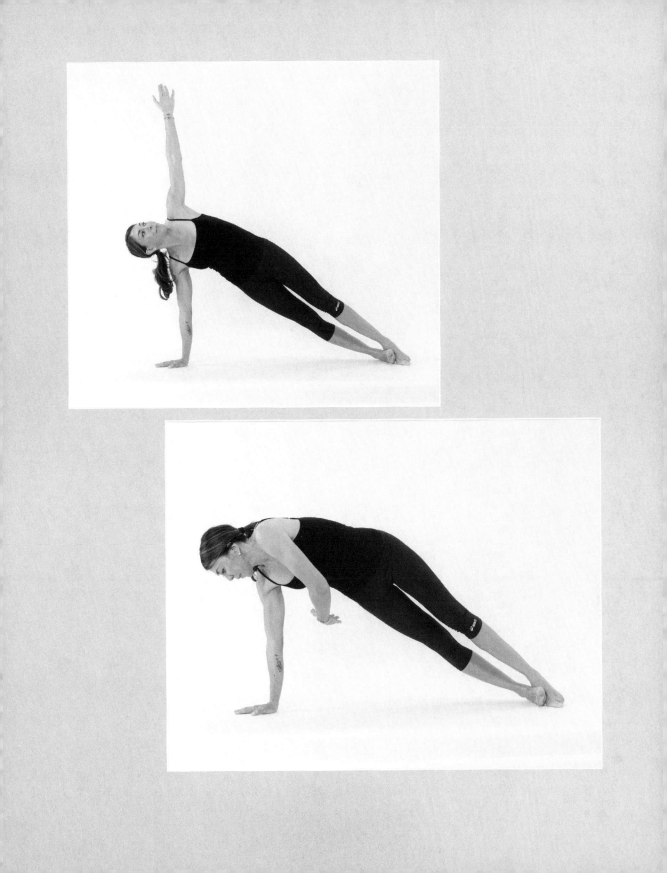

restorative yoga using props

Aproactive effort to restore the body is a critical facet of fitness training that many athletes underutilize. Unfortunately and misguidedly, we are often taught that pushing ourselves to the limits of our ability is the way to get better at our sport. But it is during rest, not during training, that we grow stronger. It allows the body to adapt to the demands placed on it through gentle stretching, massaging, and creating space in the muscles and connective tissue that have undergone stress. According to the Chinese principle of yin and yang, rest and action are interdependent: The deeper we rest, the higher we perform. Sleep is necessary but not sufficient; to encourage high achievement, athletes must supplement 8 to 10 hours of sleep with a conscious restorative practice.

This is why restorative yoga, through active and restorative poses, is an essential part of improving athletic performance. Active poses will improve postural alignment, create a greater core/center focus, "fill in" where you are not flexible, and provide a mental focal point to help you relax. For physical and mental reasons, rest is just as important as high-intensity training for success and progress in athletics. Without resting properly, you limit the extent of your performance and make yourself vulnerable to overexhaustion and injury. As with regular formats of yoga, restorative yoga poses can treat the entire body at once or target more specific areas. For example, supported relaxation helps the entire body and mind relax, while certain poses zero in on certain body parts.

These deeply relaxing poses not only encourage better posture, flexibility, and safe muscle repair; they also increase blood flow to the tendons, ligaments, and bones, which are even more susceptible to stress and overtraining. Creating relaxed synergy among muscles, fascia, and connective tissues, restorative yoga also allows your hormones to come back into balance, which helps them kick into gear more quickly and effectively during training.

Many athletes work in a constant state of fatigue because they do not give themselves enough time to assimilate their workload. The only way to make progress is to replenish your energy resources through physical restoration. Otherwise, you run the risk of strain, injury, and overtraining. By preventing these issues, restorative yoga increases your athletic life span and enjoyment of your sport.

At the elite level, an athlete's success begins to depend more on their mental game than on their physical game. Restorative yoga helps athletes develop the mental strength required for high performance. Athletic success depends partially on the ability to motivate and push but even more so on the ability to calm and focus the mind during periods of high physical stress. The meditation and mindfulness components of yoga train athletes to return to a calm mental center that they can utilize during competition to increase strength and endurance.

Restorative yoga uses props such as blankets, bands, and blocks to support and release the skeletal-muscular system in gentle positions. Props also allow you to hold poses for longer, giving you an opportunity to release tension and create space in the muscles for longer.

Props make your practice fun, lively, more work and less work, respectively, by assisting or (sometimes) resisting your poses. You can purchase the props mentioned in this book at YogaFit.com.

Restorative yoga is the ultimate cross-training tool for any sport, and I suggest you incorporate the following sequence once or twice a week after your workout. Dim the lights, set your props up, and put some relaxing music on such as YogaFit's *Peaceful Paradise* or *Music for Relaxation and Meditation* CD. Each pose can be held for up to twenty minutes at a time, so make sure to block off enough time to truly focus on your restorative practice. Breathe and restore. Restorative yoga should be used 1–2 times a week to balance the body (think cross-training) and reduce tightness and overuse injuries. If you are feeling especially tight or stressed, you should do restorative yoga more often.

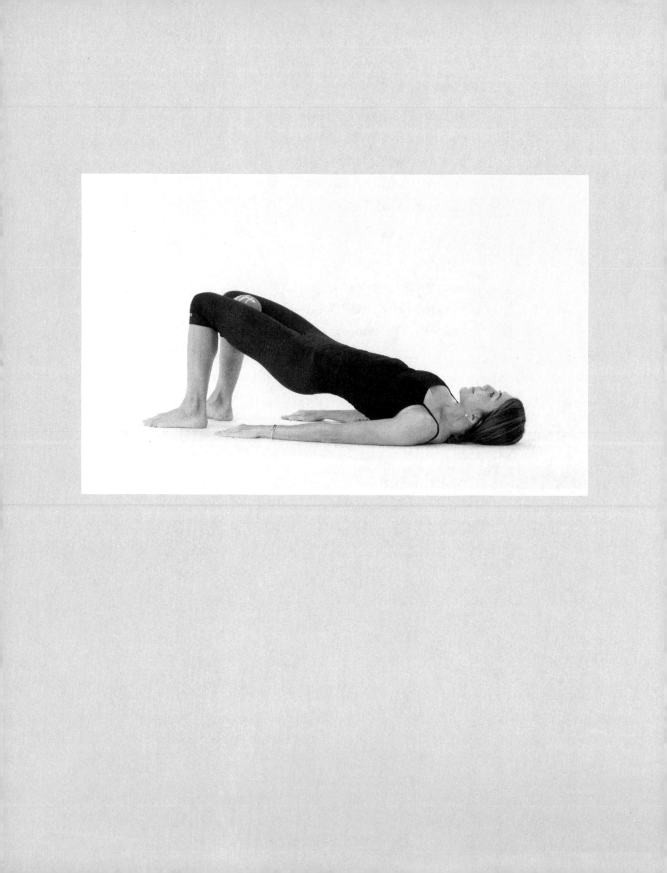

BRIDGE with EGGS or CORE BALL

Benefit of the pose: Bridge opens the front of your hips and strengthens your back and inner thighs. Having an egg between your thighs will help you activate your adductors and maintain alignment of your knees over your ankles.

Getting into the pose: Lie flat on your mat with your knees bent. Place an egg block or core ball between your thighs and leave your hands on the mat along your sides. Press into your heels to lift your pelvis toward the sky, squeezing the egg block firmly enough to hold it in place.

Holding the pose: Reach your thigh bones away from your body as you lift, maintaining equal tension throughout the back of your body. Maintain a strong core center to support your lower back and resist the urge to overextend it.

Modifications: If fatigue sets in, you can flow this pose with breath. Inhale and lift, exhale and lower to your mat. If you feel pressure at the front of your knees, make sure they are directly over your ankles.

CHEST EXPANSION with a STRAP

Benefit of the pose: A strap can keep your arms in place if interlacing your fingers behind you is not possible. The strap will help you keep your shoulders open while you stretch your chest. It also strengthens your upper back muscles. This pose is revitalizing.

Getting into the pose: From a standing position, reach your shoulders up, back, and down and open up your chest. Reach behind you and take hold of the strap in both hands. Hold the strap in your fists and turn your fists so that your palms face in.

Holding the pose: Inhale and lift your heart upward and reach through the crown of your head. Exhale and engage the core center a little more and bring your hands closer together along the strap. For more sensation, reach your hips back and sit into Chair Pose and gradually reach your arms upward so that your fists are over your shoulders but past them.

Modifications: This same stretch works from a kneeling position if that is more comfortable.

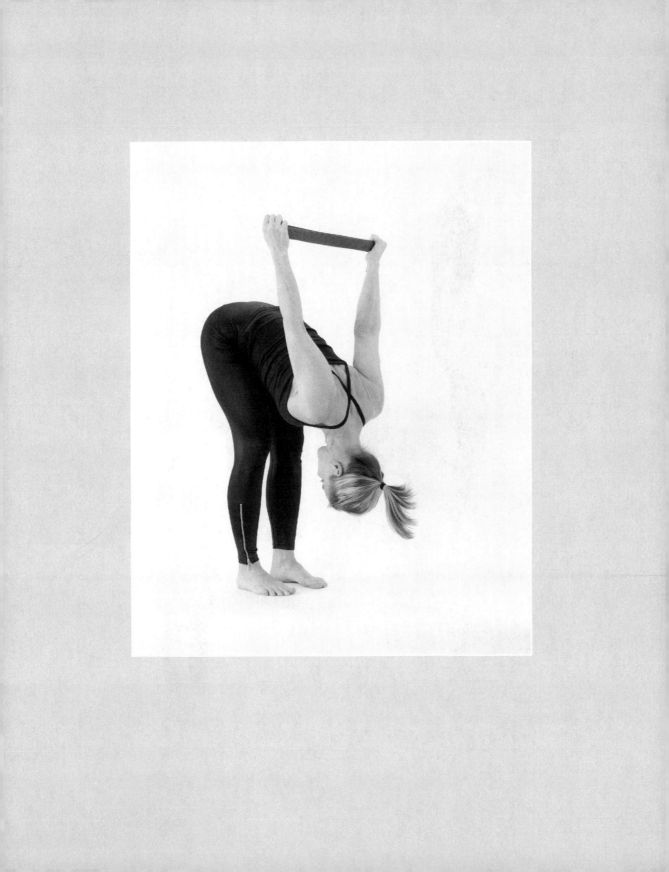

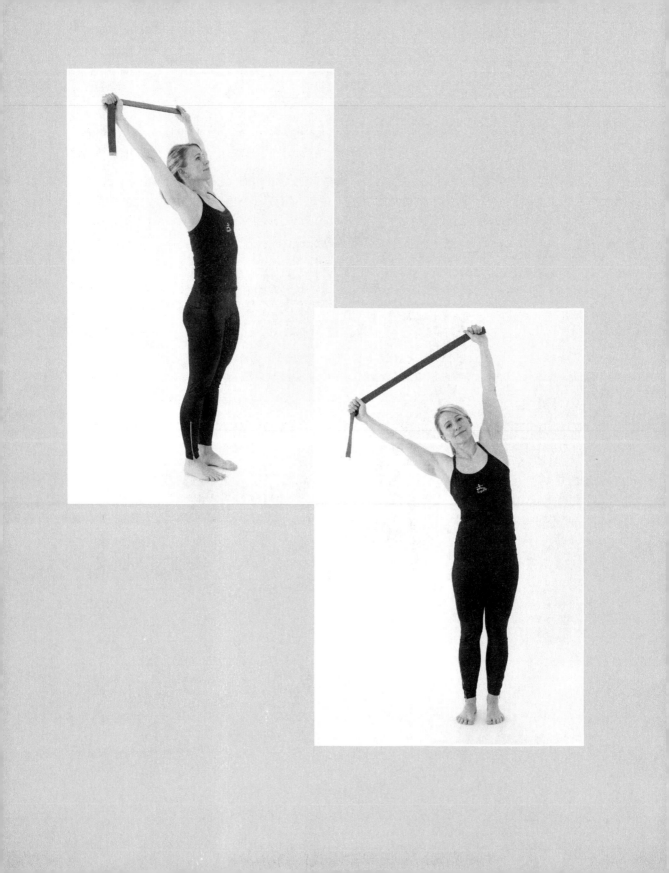

BACK BEND with a STRAP

Benefit of the pose: By holding on to the strap, you stay open in your shoulders in this pose while working your upper back muscles in a back extension. It strengthens your back muscles, as well as glutes and hamstrings, to stand strong.

Getting into the pose: Hold on to the strap in front of you, pulling gently to create tension in the strap. Stand tall, engaging your inner thighs and core center. Lengthen your spine through the crown of your head and raise your arms above you while holding the strap.

Holding the pose: Continue to stand tall and reach up and back a little further. Squeeze your inner thighs and keep your legs and body long, stretching through your chest.

Modifications: If you feel tension in your lower back, you are likely reaching back too far or not reaching up enough. Ease off the extension and reach up further.

Option to side bend: Anchor your feet to your mat and lift tall through your legs and spine. Reach above you with your hands, holding the strap while releasing through your shoulders. As you reach up, lift up and over as you flex your spine sideways. This option opens up the sides of your torso and creates core awareness.

ASSISTED HAMSTRING STRETCH

Benefit of the pose: In this pose, the strap allows you to stay upright while you hold up your leg. You can also walk your hands down the strap the longer you stay in the pose. It stretches the hamstrings on your raised leg while strengthening the hamstrings and glutes on your standing leg.

Getting into the pose: Make a small loop in the strap and place it around your foot. Lift and extend your leg off the floor. Use the strap to assist your leg upward, keeping your body upright and your spine long.

Holding the pose: Inhale and lift your body tall through the crown of your head. Exhale and draw your leg up further with the strap.

Modifications: If there is tension through the body while standing, lie on your back on your mat and do the same thing with one leg raised to the sky with the option of lowering your leg to the side.

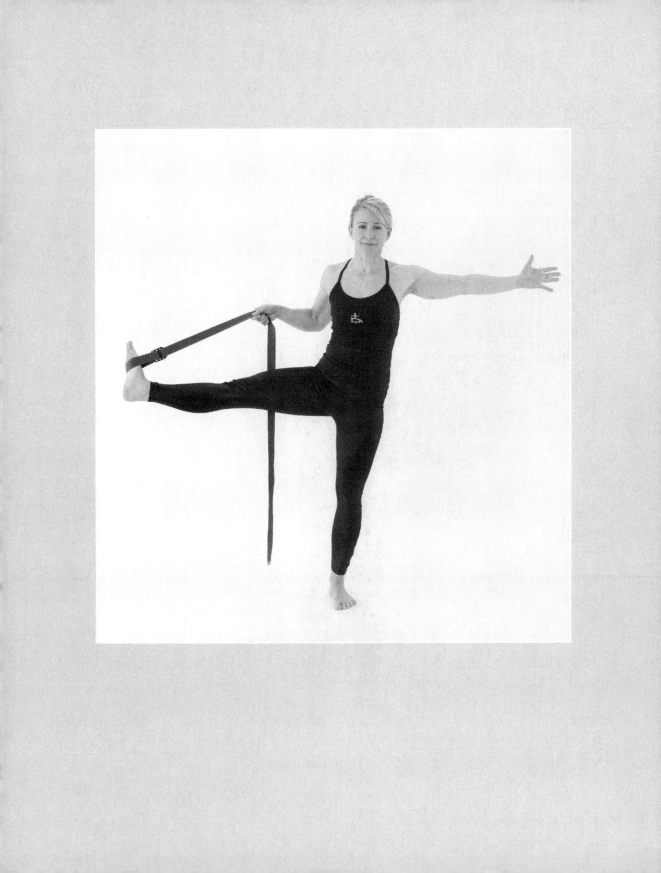

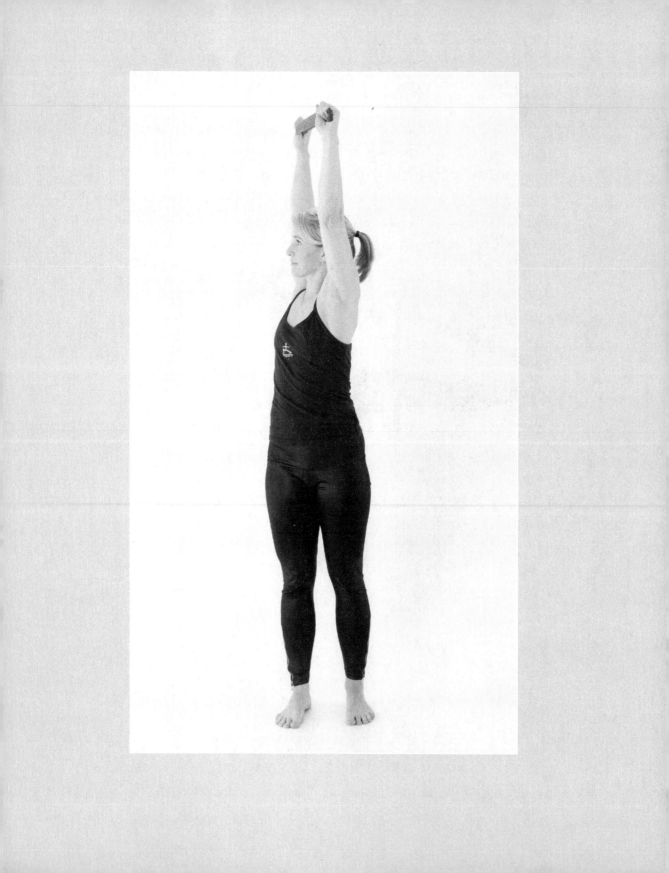

STANDING SPINAL TWIST with a STRAP

Benefit of the pose: This is essentially the standing hamstring stretch with a twist added. This stretches and strengthens your hamstrings and obliques. As mentioned, twists also massage your internal organs, and release serotonin from your gut.

Getting into the pose: Standing with both feet hip-width apart at the top of your mat, lengthen your spine and rotate toward your standing leg. Twist with your navel, chest, then shoulders and switch your hands, reaching your other arm back.

Holding the pose: Inhale and lengthen your spine to the sky. Exhale and rotate further into the twist.

Modifications: This pose can also be done on the floor. Instead of twisting toward your raised leg, bring your raised leg across your body to the other side of your mat. Keep your spine long.

FISH POSE with EGGS

Benefit of the pose: Fish Pose opens you across your chest and shoulders. The contour shape of the eggs fully supports your spine in an extended position. With this support, the body can be at rest for a more restorative approach.

Getting into the pose: From a seated position, place three egg blocks together behind you. Roll onto the rounded edge of the blocks with your upper back, not your lower back. Extend your legs along your mat and release your arms out to your sides in a comfortable position.

Holding the pose: With each exhale, release tension and become more and more relaxed. Enjoy the stillness.

Modifications: If your neck feels too extended, place another egg block under your head.

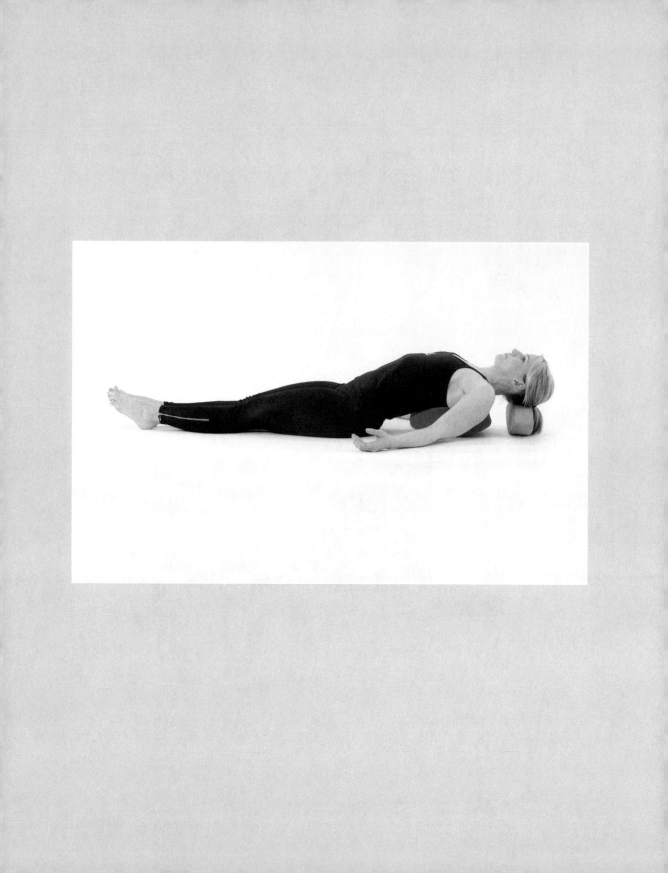

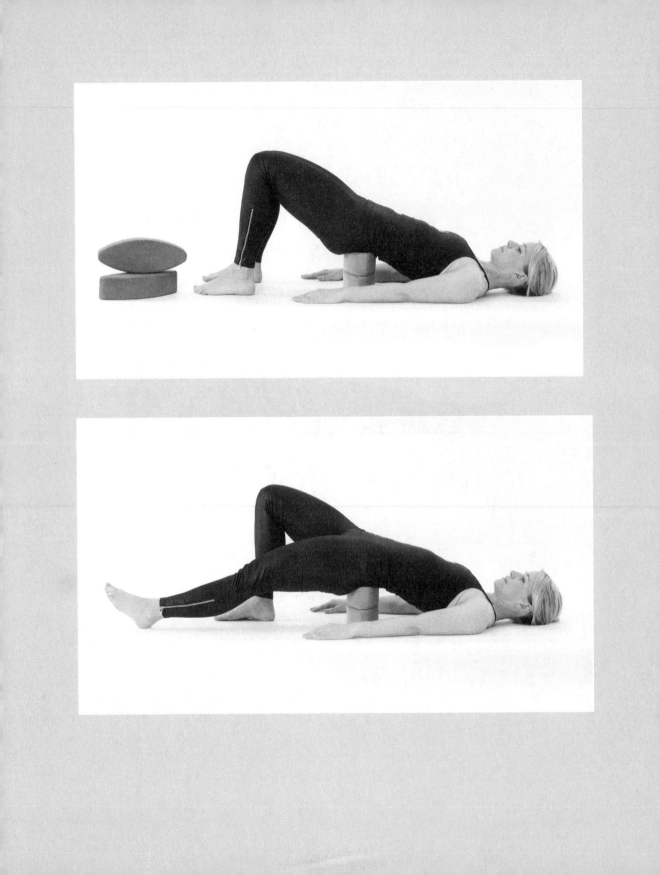

SUPPORTED BRIDGE and HIP FLEXOR STRETCH with EGGS

Benefit of the pose: This pose releases the front of your hips. The egg blocks support your hips in a raised position, and gravity releases your hips. This makes the pose more restorative because your opposing muscles—your glutes and your hamstrings—are at rest.

Getting into the pose: Lie on your back on your mat. Bend your knees and place your feet hip-width apart. Press into your feet to lift your pelvis just enough to place two egg blocks (flat sides together, stacked) under your pelvis. Lower your hips to the blocks.

Holding the pose: Release your arms to the sides, even overhead, if comfortable. Find rest through the front and back of your hips.

Modifications: If you feel tension in your lower back, then take one of the egg blocks out.

From Bridge to Hip Flexor Stretch: One side at a time, extend one leg by sliding your foot out along your mat. Relax your foot on your mat and feel the stretch in your hips, then switch sides.

LOWER BACK RELEASE

Benefit of the pose: The name of this pose explains it all. In a position lying facedown on your mat, tension is released from your lower back. This pose also aids with digestion and releases serotonin in the gut.

Getting into the pose: Place two egg blocks in the middle of your mat with the curved side up. From a kneeling position, walk your hands forward and lower your hip bones down to the block. Place the front of your hips across the block as you lower yourself.

Holding the pose: Find rest with your arms in front of you, one hand over the other. Rest your forehead or cheek on top of your hands.

Modifications: If there is discomfort in the abdomen, the block may be positioned too high along your torso. Bring it down across the pelvis. If it feels too high, use a rolled-up mat for less elevation.

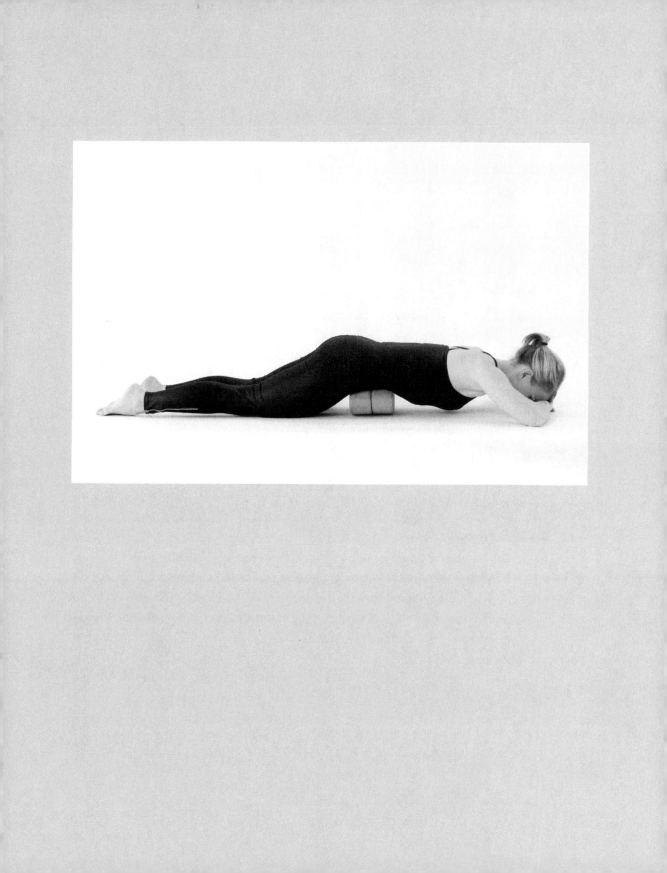

weight training with yoga

I've been working out with weights since I was fifteen, and I cannot get enough of the feeling that pumping iron provides. Combining yoga with weights marries two of the most effective approaches to fitness—improving multiple aspects of your physical health and mental well-being. Weight training with yoga infuses your workout with added calorie-burning power from the weights while providing the mentally centering benefits of traditional poses. Concentrating on yoga poses and deep breathing helps you feel peaceful and relaxed, but the extra resistance of weights helps get your heart rate up to an aerobic level.

Using 2-, 3-, 5-, or 7.5-pound weights or kettlebells in yoga challenges the body to engage its stabilizing muscles and enhance strength, flexibility, balance, and your overall level of conditioning. It increases mobility in the spine, joints, and tendons, providing an overall improvement in range of motion. By now, you understand the importance of those elements in your athletic performance and improvement.

Adding weights to your yoga practice accelerates your physical progress in yoga and helps you feel grounded. Also, as you develop an understanding of your body as it relates to your specific sport, weights will help you focus on your use of muscles in each position. Incorporating weights will quickly and effectively target specific muscle groups, helping to tone and build strength in particular areas like your arms, thighs, and abdominals.

The weight-bearing aspects of yoga can be supplemented with breathing techniques, which we cover in a later chapter, that help to oxygenate the muscles. The increased blood flow, oxygen, and delivery of nutrients make muscles less prone to strain and tear while promoting growth and repair.

Breathing heightens your awareness of movement and leads you to think about what is contracting and expanding and where you feel openness or discomfort. It's easy to lose touch with these elements of self-awareness in a regular workout and even in a yoga practice if the routine has become too familiar or repetitive. Yoga with weights renews your awareness of your body by grounding you with added resistance, bringing your attention to the details of each exercise.

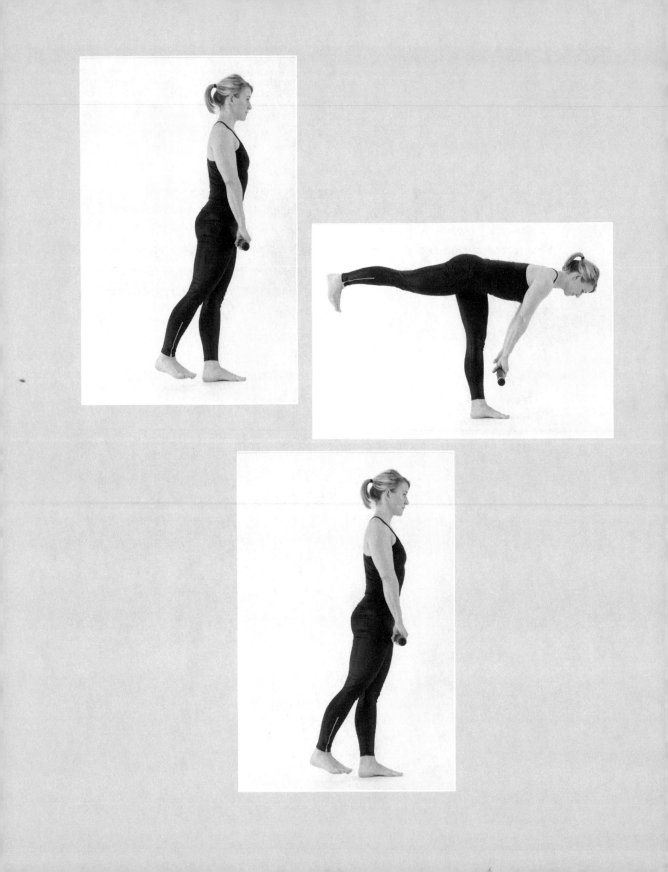

WARRIOR III to STANDING with BARBELL
(SINGLE-LEG DEADLIFT)

Benefit of the Pose: Like a common exercise in the weight room, the deadlift, when performing Warrior III to Standing you strengthen your glutes and hamstrings. With weight you get to challenge your muscles even more. Doing a single-leg deadlift allows you to focus on strength and control through your range of motion one side of your body at a time, whereas when you do both legs at once, often one side compensates for a weakness in the opposite side without your realizing it.

Getting into the pose: From Mountain, hold the bar in front of you. Stabilize your pelvis and extend one leg back. Hinge forward on your standing leg and lift your back leg simultaneously. Keep the bar right beneath your shoulders and keep your pelvis level as you lower your upper body and raise your back leg to a parallel position with the floor. With your standing leg, use strong activation through your glute and hamstring and return to standing. Keep your pelvis level and your spine long.

Modifications: It is imperative that your upper body and extended leg create one long line without any curves, especially your spine. If this is a new exercise, do the exercise without any weight to master form and then add weight when you are ready.

WARRIOR III with BARBELL ROW

Benefit of the pose: Warrior III with weight is essentially like doing a single-leg deadlift. It strengthens your glutes and hamstrings. Adding the barbell row strengthens your upper back and rear shoulders.

Getting into the pose: From a standing position, hold the bar with your hands wider than your shoulders. While you stand on one leg, extend and straighten the other leg back. Keep your back leg straight as your torso hinges over your standing leg until you are parallel to the floor. Keep your leg and torso straight and bring the bar to your chest and lower. Hold your leg and torso in this position while you continue to row the bar. Repeat 12–15 times.

Modifications: If you notice tension or if your back rounds, use less weight to start and work up to more. You could also use a strap to simulate a barbell row. Hang on to the strap at either end. Create tension in the strap and pull the strap to your chest.

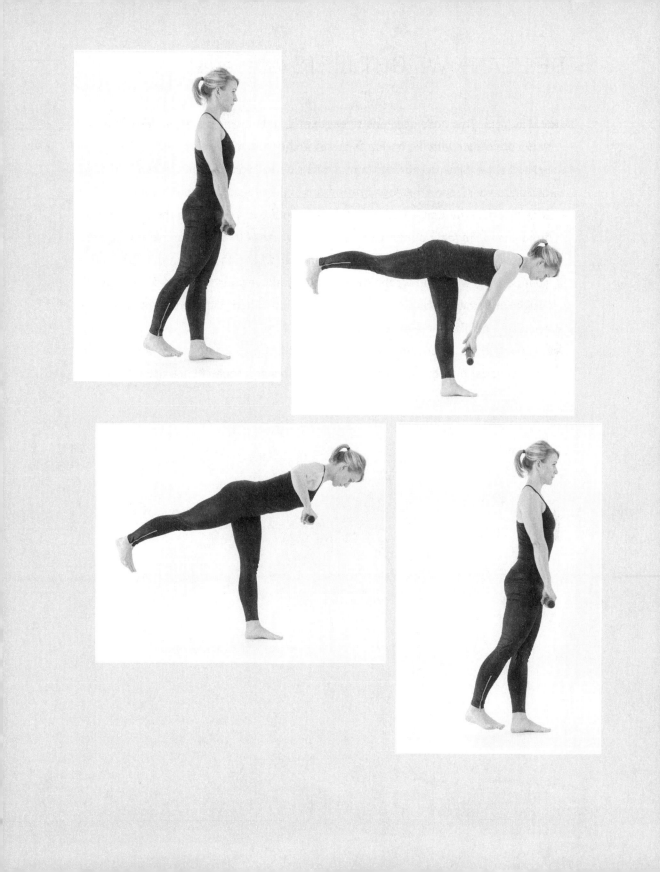

SIDE PLANK WEIGHT LIFTS (20–30 REPS)

Benefit of the pose: This pose develops strength and stability in your shoulders, hips, and your core center with the option to increase the work with weight.

Getting into the pose: Sit with your legs bent to one side and your top knee raised so that you can place your feet on the floor, one in front of the other. Place your hand on the floor directly under your shoulder and stabilize. Hold the weight with the other hand in front of you. Engage your core center and lengthen your spine from your tailbone to the crown of your head. Press into your foot and hand that are on the floor and lift your body up while you lift the weight directly above your shoulder. Then lower the weight underneath you while you keep your hips lifted. Lift the weight above your shoulder again and repeat 20–30 times.

Modifications: If there is tension in your shoulders, bring your forearm to your mat with your shoulder directly over your elbow. You can also choose Kneeling Side Plank.

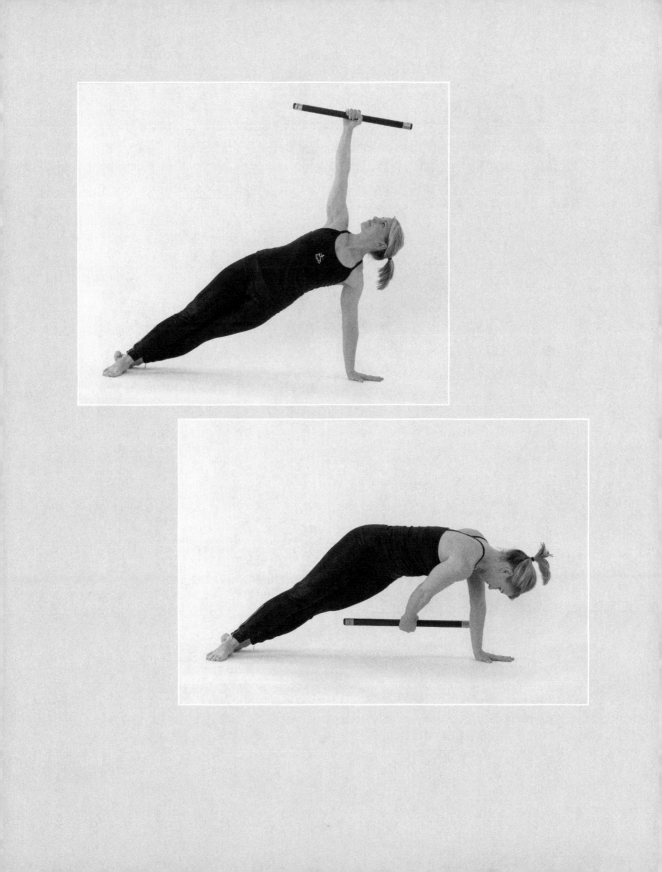

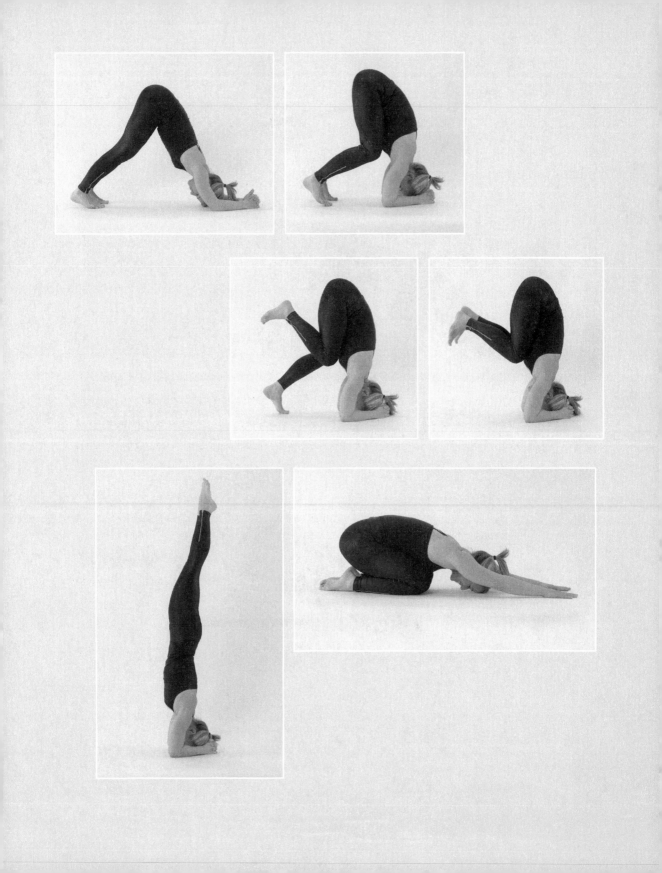

FOREARM BALANCE

Benefit of the Pose: You are essentially using the weight of your entire body to build strength in your shoulders and upper back. It also builds strength in your hips and core center to control the lift of your legs. It requires an incredible amount of strength, stability, and focus to execute this posture. As an inversion, blood flow to your brain increases.

CAUTION: As a beginner, do this pose in front of a wall to prevent you from falling backward. Proper warmup (Chair Flow p. 30, Half Series p. 40) is mandatory, and prep work (Dolphin Pose p. 75, Core and Balance Poses p. 240) is highly recommended for your safety. This pose is not recommended for anyone with head, neck, eye, or spine injuries.

Getting into the pose: Kneel in front of a wall and place your hands about a hand's distance away and come down to your forearms, as in Dolphin Pose. Wrap your hands around the outside of your elbows to ensure that your elbows are directly under your shoulders, then return your forearms to the floor. Interlace your fingers except your pinkies; place them one in front of the other. Stabilize your shoulders and walk your feet inward, using tiptoes if necessary. Lift your hips high, keeping as much of your upper body over your shoulders as possible. Bring your feet off the floor one at a time by bending one knee and then the other. When you are ready to come down, gently tuck your knees in and place your toes then knees to the floor and rest in Child's Pose.

Holding the pose: Breathe and focus on your whole body. Lengthen your tailbone upward to the sky, keeping your spine long even with your legs tucked. Work to stabilize with your hips lifted and your knees in a tucked position.

Taking it further: Once you are stable, begin to lift your legs slowly. Focus on steady movement and breathe while you lift your legs until fully extended. Use the wall intermittently, if required, as you lift your legs.

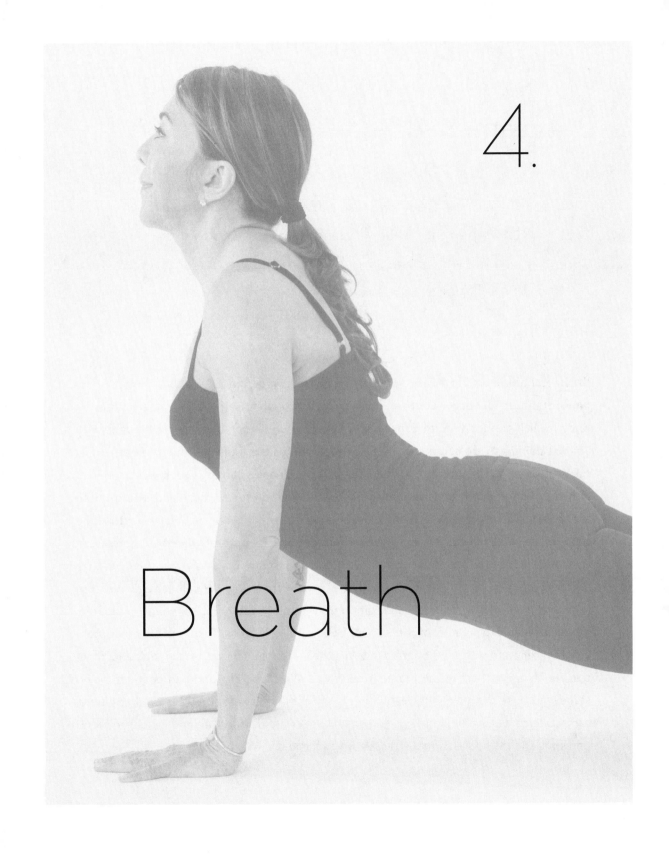

4.

Breath

breath

When the breath wanders, the mind also is unsteady.
But when the breath is calmed the mind too will be still,
and the yogi achieves long life. Therefore, one should
learn to control the breath.

—**Svatmarama**, *Hatha Yoga Pradipika*

Breath control is vital to athletic performance. When you control your breathing you enhance your focus, concentration, and discipline. Thích Nhất Hạnh says, "The breath is the bridge which connects life to consciousness, which unites the body to the thoughts." In YogaFit trainings we say it more simply: "Breath unites the body and mind." Breathing is the pathway to mindfulness, clarity, and physical awareness. Learning to control your breath enhances energy, increases metabolism, and will allow you to feel, heal, and be present to the moment. Learning how to breathe deeply, both on and off your mat, can clear the loud noise of life and can help reduce or even eliminate some symptoms triggered by stress.

If you want to win you must perform well, and to perform optimally you must visualize and become present with what your body and breath are doing. We will delve deeper into the benefits of meditation and visualization next, but first you must learn how to breathe. We all know how to breathe, of course. Our bodies innately do it; it's something that occurs automatically and without thought. However, there are many things that restrict and affect our breathing, not just in the moment but habitually. Slouching and bad posture, for instance, collapse the lungs and restrict a healthy pathway; stress, pressure, and emotions can create convulsive breathing patterns that trigger rapid heart rate and increased blood pressure; and muscle tension distresses the inhale and exhale patterns.

When playing sports, you're taught to "keep your eye on the ball"; when you breathe consciously, you're taught to keep your third eye (or "inner eye," meaning the passage of wisdom) focused on your breath. Tapping into your breath and using it as a tool to calm and relax will strengthen your focus and concentration.

Envision yourself in a high-stress moment. The clock is ticking down, you're flustered because you can't find an open teammate, and you start to panic. Your breath becomes quick and wayward, and all of a sudden your stress level has increased, your concentration is cloudy, and you've lost focus. The stress is already there—in the clock, in the stands, in the internal voice—but if you can truly find a way to calm yourself by controlling and calming your breath, the external noise will begin to diminish.

Yoga practitioners have incorporated breathing practices for years, because they understood the correlation between steady, controlled breath and mental and physical vitality. Modern science agrees that if your breath is out of control, fast, and shallow, it can cause a slew of problems, including fatigue, sleep disorders, anxiety, heartburn, muscle cramps, dizziness, visual problems, chest pain, and heart palpitations. So what does controlled breath do, and how do you do it?

Let's begin with its effect on the steady flow of oxygen. Breath is the only means of supplying our organs with oxygen, which is vital for our health and survival, and it helps rid our bodies of waste products and toxins.

Oxygen purifies the bloodstream and aids in the proper functioning of the brain, nerves, glands, and other internal organs. Most important, it gives your organs the energy and rejuvenation they need to thrive. If your body is starved for oxygen, your blood is affected. A hunger for oxygen is caused by quick and shallow breathing. Through the slow and steady nature of yoga, you tap into this vital nutrient and center yourself on a sound flow of breath from one pose to the next. The key here is translating those breath patterns off the mat and into your game.

Mentally, steady breath will positively affect your well-being as it cleanses, focuses, and relaxes the mind. If your breathing fluctuates in any way, whether through shortness or quickness of breath, it will trigger your psyche to react. When you take a moment to slow your breath, your respiratory system is calmed, as is your heart rate. When I work with NFL officials, I notice that when they have controlled breath it makes them concentrated on the field, rather than their surroundings, and gives them a one-pointed presence. Referees receive a lot of flak, especially in high-pressure situations such as the playoffs, as their decisions can potentially affect the outcome of the game. One call can mean a win or a loss, and having the ability to concentrate fully and avoid stress getting in the way is important. Focusing on the breath helps those referees relax, which leads to a better and more poised performance.

The Effects of Shallow Breathing

- Reduced oxygen: With a reduction in circulating oxygen you lose energy and vitality.
- Susceptibility to disease: Oxygen is essential to produce healthy cells. It is possible to catch more colds and develop other ailments more easily if your breath is hindered.
- Diminished mental ability can occur because tension in the brain is produced by restricted breathing.

Where to Begin?

The nose. Breathing through your nose rather than your mouth gives you a sense of control, and it is also a natural defense mechanism that wards off germs. Those pesky nose hairs? We have them for a reason. They are actually little warriors that block dust and particles from entering your body and injuring your lungs. The nose also leads to a passageway lined with mucus membranes that warms cold air and catches outside elements. The mouth, in general, cannot guard from harmful matter that sneaks its way into our bodies through breathing.

Ancient yogis also credit the nose with absorbing free energy (also known as *prana*), and they believe that the physical, mental, emotional, and spiritual effects of right and left nostril breathing relate to the movement of the prana through the nostrils (*nadas*). The logic goes that right nostril breath is the warming or stimulating breath used to increase energy or alertness and the left nostril has the opposite effects.

Safe Breathing Tips

- Consult your physician prior to advanced breathing techniques or breath suspension.
- Learn your favorite breathing practice and do it outside in the morning when the air is fresh.
- Wear loose, non-restrictive clothing.
- Avoid areas with polluted air, including rooms with smoke from candles and incense.
- If you are sick or have asthma, lung issues, or heart disease, refrain.
- If you are pregnant, avoid Breath of Fire and Breath Suspension.
- Avoid suspending your breath if you have high blood pressure—it can temporarily raise your blood pressure.
- Stop if you feel dizzy or lightheaded.
- Remain relaxed throughout the entire breath exercise.

Guided Practice

The techniques in this book are a few of my favorites that you can incorporate into your daily life. *Pranayama*, also known as the practice of breath control, consists of a series of exercises that guide concentration, meditation, and physical connection or oneness. The following four practices will improve your athletic performance, cultivate a general sense of clarity through life, and improve your oxygen intake for a healthier body.

MEASURED, FOCUSED BREATHING

These are simple breaths that calm the mind and help you get present and focused.

1. **Lying down if possible, spread your hands across your belly with your thumbs touching your lower ribs and your pinky fingers at your hip bones. Inhale a count of 8, hold for 8, then exhale.**

2. While you are breathing, focus your attention on the spot between your eyebrows. This is known as the third eye. The third eye is the center of your insight and intuition, and focusing on it instead of the distractions around you—the taunting, hissing, music, and so on—will help you be the best at your game.

Prescription: Practice this for 5–15 minutes or when you need to reduce anxiety and get focused, perhaps before a match or game.

BREATH OF FIRE

When you wake up or when you're getting ready for your workout, this breath warms up the body, revs up your metabolism, and helps calm the mind and burn away distractions.

This practice uses deep, rapid breath cycles to warm your body and to increase your energy. Traditionally, the breath of fire is not a pranayama technique but rather a *kriya*, or cleansing, practice. Many of the toxins in your body are released during your exhale, which is the focus here.

1. Find a comfortable seated or reclining position.
2. Keeping your mouth closed, begin inhaling through your nose.
3. Exhale half the air out of your lungs to a point somewhere between exhale and inhale.
4. Your exhale should be quick and sharp, contracting your abdominal muscles. In this exercise, exhalations are short, vigorous, and active, while inhalations are light and passive.
5. Continue this rhythmic pattern for 20–25 breaths. Repeat 2–5 rounds, finishing with a deep three-part breath.

The key for this breathing technique is to fully expand the belly with the breath and fully empty it out.

> One way to start Breath of Fire is with long, deep breathing. As soon as your lungs are completely expanded, as described earlier, immediately force the air out. Once most of it is out, immediately expand the air back in, each time arching your spine forward and pressing your palms inward against your knees in a light manner to feel your diaphragm. Fill your lungs from the back to the front completely, contracting repeatedly.

Prescription: Three rounds with a hold of the breath in between. Try to do Breath of Fire on all fours and watch your belly fill and contract.

ALTERNATE NOSTRIL BREATHING

This technique balances the right and left hemispheres of the brain to calm and energize. It is said in Ayurveda and in the therapeutic yoga tradition that alternate nostril breathing can be helpful for equalizing the activity in the right and left hemispheres of the brain while relaxing the nervous system and calming the mind. When we do alternate nostril breathing, we literally switch which nostril we breathe in and out of in a rhythmic pattern.

1. Do a simple breath focus exercise to start (close your eyes and take ten deep breaths, focusing on how your body feels and scanning your body for any pain, injury, or special conditions, as well as parts of your body that feel energized), then raise your right hand to your face with your palm facing in.

2. Using your right hand with your fingers outstretched, block off your right nostril by putting gentle pressure on it with your thumb. Be sure to keep the rest of your fingers straight and pointing up toward the sky. Your fingers act like antennas for more energy.

3. With a long, slow, deep breath, gently inhale through your left nostril. Then release your thumb and, using the index finger of your right hand, block off your left nostril and exhale long, slowly, and completely, through your right nostril.

4. **Keeping your left nostril blocked with your index finger, inhale slowly and fully through your right nostril.**

5. **Switch your fingers again so that your right thumb is blocking your right nostril and exhale completely through your left nostril.**

6. **Continue to alternate with one complete inhale/exhale per thumb/finger.**

Prescription: 5–10 minutes

BREATH SUSPENSION

> One does not simply hold the breath by physical retention, but holds on to the very self, which was raised up and elated through the inhalation.
>
> —B.K.S. Iyengar

Suspending the breath helps integrate the body systems, helps assimilate the energy just created in your pranayama (and asana). Breath Suspension can give you a tremendous sense of peace and calmness.

Suspending on the inhale:

- Inhale to the lungs' full capacity.
- Lift your upper ribs, and tuck your chin—your shoulders, throat, and face should be relaxed.
- You are not holding on to the breath in tension, but simply allowing it to be suspended in the lungs.
- You become still and calm.

- Sometimes if you sip in a bit more air when you feel that urge to exhale, you can suspend a little longer.

Suspending on the exhale:

- Exhale all air out of your lungs.
- Draw your belly button toward your spine, lift your diaphragm, compress your upper chest, and tuck your chin.
- Become still and calm.
- Exhale a bit more air to lengthen the time of suspension.

5.

Visualization,
Guided Imagery,
and Meditation

> Shuniya is a deep stillness, into which you can plant a seed—bij—to create a new rhythm or pattern of being. In shuniya the Kundalini flows.
>
> —Yogi Bhajan

Yoga, in all of its parts, unites the body and mind to create a well-balanced life. Through the physical yoga poses, you strengthen your overall functionality for better performance and agility. Through controlled breathing, you learn to calm your nervous system and improve your focus. Now, we will look at the mental aspect of yoga that teaches you how to use your mind as a powerful tool to form positivity, realize goals, and quell your stressful thoughts. With guided imagery, you will train and positively direct your performance to improve, while visualization and meditation will teach focus and clarity in order to achieve greatness and an overall state of calm. The pressure of an athlete can be mentally straining, but learning how to dispose of the negativity and outside burdens will lead you to more dedicated training and a higher concentration in and out of the game.

Your mind is a powerful tool—it can trick you, and it can guide you. For instance, if you feel an itch in your throat and you begin to dwell on that feeling of sickness, oftentimes the fixation you create becomes your mind and body's main focus. That worry can actually lead you to becoming sick. Stress disturbs your entire nervous system; if you allow it to take over with destructive thoughts, your entire body will be affected. If you are able to master your thoughts and guide them to success, your mind will be your most valued asset.

Mental training is as important as, if not more important than, physical training because you will not achieve your personal physical best without the proper mindset. It is my intention that you become your own coach so that you can continue being supported and encouraged off the field. You know better than anyone else which mental, physical, and technical aspects of your game or event need work. Therefore, you are more likely to carry out your own advice than someone else's.

Dr. William J. Kroger, author of the most comprehensive textbook on hypnosis, *Clinical and Experimental Hypnosis* (written in 1963), observed that the individual is more willing to respond to his or her own suggestions. When a person suggests thoughts to himself or herself, this is much more meaningful than when they are given to him or her by someone else. It may also be unlikely that your coach will know much about the variety of mental training strategies, the many types of meditation, or the use of hypnosis or visualization. So to properly prepare yourself mentally, it is best to develop and draw on your own resources.

Across the board, humanity has conceptualized visualization as a tool to accomplish greatness. The Taoists say that there is no difference between dreaming and being awake. In one of my favorite songs, R. Kelly emphasizes that "if you can dream it, you can be it," and one of my favorite paintings by Peter Tunny has the quote, "nothing happens, unless first a dream."

It's a natural part of the human condition to value goals, dreams, and desires. As an athlete, whether you are a professional or a weekend warrior, goals are paramount to success. In life and work, success begins with a goal—completing a marathon, losing weight, asking for a raise, or giving up alcohol. Big or small, a goal gives you purpose and acts like a compass to keep you moving in the right direction. It will inspire you to wake up every day, and dreams keep you reaching for creative and inspired aspirations.

Over two thousand years ago, Aristotle spoke of achieving goals: "First, have a definite, clear, practical ideal; a goal, an objective. Second, have the necessary means to achieve your ends: wisdom, money, materials, and methods. Third, adjust all your means to that end."

Many goals stay at the "setting stage" but never progress, and we see this a lot with goals relating to physical activity and weight loss, especially around the New Year. We start out with good intentions and a plan, but then we can't seem to make it happen. The *big* question is, how do we not only improve discipline but excel at the sport or activity (work) of our choice? Mind over matter.

For the purpose of visualization and understanding the power the mind holds, I created the idea of "The Winner's Coin," a practical tool I want you to use to aid your thoughts. As with any coin, there are two sides—one side is where you will practice visualization and guided imagery. This side is filled with positivity and possibility that you will use to envision the things you want to achieve in your sport. Is it a championship ring? A hole in one? Beating your personal record? That side of the coin is for you to hold those images.

On the other is an empty space that, during meditation, you will use to place negativity and excuses along with your burdens and adverse thoughts: "I'm not good enough," "I'll never be able to slam dunk," and so on.

Learning to discipline your mind to focus on one thing (or one side) at a time will benefit you in all areas of your life. You're certainly allowed to honor your negative thoughts, but what I want you to do is learn how to let go of them so that they do not become your main focus. It is my goal to teach you how to visualize your goals and then actualize them.

In relationships, work, or studies, you will benefit from this technique, but in your sport, you will especially grow during training and competition by putting your mind on the game or movement rather than the audience's taunts and pressures. For any of the following techniques I highly suggest doing *both* guided imagery and visualization, on the one hand, and meditation, on the other, every day to create a habit. All of these tools are like going to a gym for the mind. And just like any gym experience, you must go often and keep going. Repetition creates new neural pathways, but it does not happen overnight. Keep flexing your mental muscles with daily meditation, guided imagery, and positive self-talk affirmations.

visualization and guided imagery

Just as I said in my bestselling book *YogaLean*, diet is 75 percent of staying fit, and it's been said that athletic success is 90 percent mental and 10 percent physical. When split-seconds or centimeters define a champion, having a mental edge can be crucial, which is why many athletes turn to mental imagery to take their game to the next level. The concept of mental imagery includes the mental practice of performance skills, confidence and positive thinking, problem solving, anxiety control, performance analysis, preparation, and mental clarity.

Before you can believe in a goal, you first must have an idea of what it looks like. This is where visualization comes in; it's a technique for creating a mental image of a future event. When you visualize your desired outcome, you begin to "see" the possibility of achieving it. Through visualization, you catch a glimpse of your "preferred future." When this happens, you are motivated and prepared to pursue your goal.

Visual imagery works because you imagine yourself at your peak performance and your ideal state. It's rare that you drift into a daydream where you visualize and hope that your team loses a game because of you. Through repetitive visualizations, you are creating neural pathways in the brain, clusters of cells that work together to create memories or learned behaviors. Mental imagery trains your mind to create the neural patterns in your brain that teach your muscles to do exactly what you want them to do. All of this occurs without actually performing the physical activity, yet it achieves a similar result.

Studies show that visualization increases athletic performance by improving motivation, coordination, and concentration. It also aids in relaxation and helps reduce fear and anxiety. Imagining yourself performing an action is like a mental rehearsal meant to manifest into the future action. Countless sports legends such as Michael Jordan, Larry Bird, and Tiger Woods as well as many Olympian athletes have also used visualization to improve their performance and achieve their personal best.

Remember, you don't have to be an elite athlete to benefit from visualization. Whether you're a student, businessperson, parent, or spouse, visualization will keep you tethered to your goal and increase your chances of achieving it. The power of visualization is available to everyone.

How to Practice Visualization and Mental Imagery

There are many ways to implement visualization, and you can do it practically anywhere, on or off the field. You can practice while sitting up, lying down, or in complete silence. In a moment during a sporting event, you can take a second to visualize an action—for instance, a soccer player can use the moments before a corner kick to imagine the exact outcome, or a quarterback can throw the pass in his mind prior to calling a play. More specific guided visualizations are designed for a quiet environment before competition. In order for it to work, visualization needs to become a habit for you, so practice it when and where you can!

Try this: If your goal is to complete your first 10K race, visualize yourself crossing the finish line in the time you desire. Hold that mental image as long as possible. What are you wearing, how will your clothes feel? What does your breathing feel like? What does it feel like to pass under the finishing banner, looking at your watch with the cool air on your overheated body? Who is there to greet you as you finish? Are you running with friends?

Imagine the excitement and joy you will experience as you complete your goal. Just the thought will boost your confidence. Repeat this thought daily, and eventually you will turn that image into a reality.

meditation

There are many different types of meditation, and you can use several to enhance your performance or just one. For the purposes of this book, we will focus on just a few primary techniques.

Let's go back to The Winner's Coin. If you use one side to gather visual goals and guided imagery (your mind, your life, your game), you can flip the coin and use it during meditation to dispose of the negative feelings that bring you down. It's been said that we have, on average, about sixty thousand thoughts a day. Chances are, not all of them are positive!

Some of us, if not all of us, suffer from thoughts of self-doubt and self-criticism. When you are trying to achieve a goal, these negative thought patterns can undermine even your best efforts. I liken meditation to giving your brain and mind a shower. With a proper meditation technique you will be able to cleanse your mind, resetting and restarting it to a more peaceful, calm, and centered place. Operating from this place is an essential part of achieving your goals. When thinking about ways to increase discipline, we must all look at how we consciously or subconsciously sabotage ourselves. Meditation gives you a competitive edge as it allows the conscious and subconscious to merge.

Let's take a look at the structure of our brain so that you can see how meditation taps into and massages each aspect to enhance compassion and clarity and to create a sense of calm and centeredness in your everyday.

- **Lateral prefrontal cortex:** This is the part of the brain that is in charge of assessment. It helps you take a look at things from rational and logical perspectives and overrides bad behaviors and habits by editing your emotional response to things.
- **Medial prefrontal cortex:** This is where your brain refers to your past experiences and where you relate your personal perspective on things. It processes information that is you-specific, such as self-reflection, planning for the future, social engagement, and the feeling of empathy. Oftentimes, this part of the brain can halt you in a moment because it allows you to ruminate and worry through moments of reflection.
- **Insula:** This part monitors the feelings in your body as they relate to emotional "gut feelings" or sensations in which you respond, "Is this dangerous?"
- **Amygdala:** The alarm system of the brain, responsible for emotional reactions and responses.

Prior to meditating and soothing the neural connections in the brain, the brain will often rely on one part to delegate what is going on. If you meditate on a regular basis and tap into the workings of your mind and body, several things happen to the brain to help improve this teamwork. First, the physical feelings connected to fear and anxiety (insula) will begin to separate themselves from one another, because you will begin differentiating (and *feeling*) the truth in your physical responses. When you understand that the tingling sensation is a direct result of your emotions rather than an actual physical ailment, your anxiety begins to decrease because you're not worried about that physical feeling being something bigger than what it really is.

Also, meditation will help strengthen the lateral prefrontal cortex so that you will better understand when something is upsetting you, physically and emotionally. For instance, if you experience any level of pain, meditation will help you learn to take a step back and analyze the pain first rather than assume that something is severely wrong.

Through meditation, your brain is changed so that you can not only see yourself in a more concise perspective but the world around you too. You will begin to react in a more balanced way to the events in your life, including stressful sporting events or practices. In order to keep this steady flow, however, you must practice meditation on a regular basis because your brain, like any muscle, needs to be worked out, and without its "exercise" it will revert back to its former structure.

For athletes specifically, meditation has a slew of benefits. Consider the example of Phil Jackson, possibly the most successful coach in basketball history (eleven NBA championships). Jackson has used some rather uncommon tactics to help create these championship teams. The key and differentiating concept he employs is the idea of "building mental muscle" with "one breath, one mind," a Zen principle he implemented carefully with the Chicago Bulls. "I approach everything with mindfulness, much as we pump iron and we run to build our strength up, we need to build mental strength up . . . so we can focus . . . so the team can be in concert with one another."

One way Jackson had his team practice mindfulness was through meditation. He taught body awareness to his players—how to hold their hands, where their shoulders had to be, the whole process of being in an upright stance. He also used to teach them to play in silence and darkness on occasion to cut out all of the chatter and heighten their awareness and concentration.

Transcendental Meditation (TM) was created in 1955 by Maharishi Mahesh Yogi, who began publicly teaching a traditional meditation technique learned from his master Brahmananda Saraswati.

TM provides the experience of "restful alertness," which reduces stress, strengthens communication between the brain's prefrontal cortex and different areas of the brain, and develops total brain functioning. As a result, the TM practitioner displays stronger executive functions, with more purposeful thinking and far-sighted decision making.

Below is a list of the benefits of meditation:

- **Peak Performance**

Meditation can program your body to perform with better precision by making you better at your desired skill set. Being in an optimum state of mind will make a difference in your sport, and meditating will make you a better athlete. If you want to get the most out of your training and create conditions for excellence in athletic precision, you need to meditate.

- **Focus**

Your focus will determine if you win or lose the game. When you're not focused at the free throw line, you may miss the shot. Why not train your mind to focus? Meditation increases states of focus within the brain. Every athlete, no matter what sport they are playing, could benefit by work on their focus.

- **Pain Management and Immune System**

Most fitness instructors and professional athletes have injuries and are always dealing with some sort of pain. High-endurance sports are hard on the body, and none of us can afford to be sick. Meditation refreshes, energizes, and heals your body by healing the mind so that you can perform with more power and ease and recover more quickly and easily from any strain or old injury. I have personally meditated my way out of sprained ankles and migraines!

- **Reduces Fear, Stress, and Negativity**

Fears can hijack our minds from the present moment, and that can lead to many errors in sports. Meditation calms the amygdala even when you're not meditating. Meditation allows you to cultivate a calm center. In other words, it gets you into "the zone." Athletes are always under stress. They pride themselves on their ability to function in a high-stress environment. Ever lose a game or miss the game-winning shot? Ever fail hard? We all have, but with the proper mentality we can bounce back. Sometimes it's hard to bounce back, because we run obsessive thoughts through our minds. Meditation reduces rumination and resets our mind to focus on the present.

- **Improves Mood, Sleep, and Resiliency**

The greatest athletes in the world are the most resilient. Meditation helps you detach yourself from the negative thoughts that keep you from achieving your goals. People with more mindful traits are better able to stabilize their emotions and have better control over their moods. The competitive nature of all athletes causes them to have to deal with a roller coaster of different emotions. Meditation and then sleep can be very healing. One night of lost sleep could lose a championship; quality sleep is one of the most valuable things every athlete needs. Meditation and meta-naps can help (see below for more on meta-naps).

guided practice

Mantra-Based Meditation: The Winner's Phrase

Mantra-based meditation is my favorite type of meditation because it's easy to practice and accessible to most everyone.

> Being awakened or enlightened is not simply a mental state.
>
> It is a physiological state as well. How we breathe, how the glands secrete, how the nervous system is operating, all of this changes based on what we speak, what we hear, and what we perceive.
>
> —Yoga Bhajan

The word *mantra* means "instrument of thought," which can mean a speech, sacred text, prayer, or song of praise that meditators use as an "object" of focus. Your own personal mantra or "Winner's Phrase" can be any word or combination of words that you can repeat during your meditation. It may be something as simple as "Stay calm."

Many people have found that very quickly after taking up a mantra-based meditation, they notice a change in the quality of their lives. The mantra you choose becomes your main source of concentration and can help to still the mind. Most of our sixty thousand thoughts a day are concerned with things we fear or crave or things that irritate us or make us depressed. We naturally reduce our craving, worries, anger, and despondence when we're reciting a mantra because it helps redirect the mind. Even if there is a parallel stream of thoughts going on at the same time as the mantra, the repetition creates a sense of continuity within our experience that can grow with practice.

How to Mantra Meditate

•   Sit upright or align your spine against a wall or lie down comfortably. I like to cover my eyes with a scarf, or you can use a towel.

•   Repeat your mantra or Winner's Phrase out loud for 1–2 minutes.

•   Then bring your phrase into your inner voice and repeat over and over for 10–20 minutes.

Your Winner's Phrase becomes your mental vocal (and focal) point. Think about driving your car down the road—you need to stay focused on the road in front of you (your Winner's Phrase), but you are still aware of the rearview mirror and what's happening on each side of the car (your thoughts). Stay focused on your Winner's Phrase.

The sound of the mantra is a mental object, and paying attention to the sound of the mantra can be a form of meditation, just as paying attention to the sensations of the breath is a meditation. By bringing the mind back over and over again to the mantra, the mind can become more unified and less scattered. We become more attentive and present.

5-4-3-2-1-Meditation

This powerful meditation incorporates sound (counting) and visualization (watching the numbers) so that you get a double benefit of visual and audio influences, making the focus benefits even stronger.

- Stand or sit comfortably, close your eyes and relax.
- Place your hands on your midsection.
- Inhale and exhale naturally and begin to count your breaths, moving down a number each time you exhale until you get to 1. When you get to 1, start again at 5.
- Visualize the numbers floating about 12–15 inches in front of you. Most people find their thoughts taking them away from the counting after only a few numbers. There's nothing wrong with that. Simply start again from 1 with renewed intent to focus on your breathing and your numbers. Take it slow, relax, and be watchful.
- Repeat.

This technique can be done on the field or before the game.

Meta-naps

For those of you with sleep disorders, a meta-nap is a great way to find deep, restful, and healing sleep. *Meta-nap* is a term I coined because I used to fall asleep during my meditations. I would meditate for twenty minutes, then nap for anywhere between ten and forty minutes. When I awoke I would feel incredibly refreshed and rejuvenated. I often use meta-naps to drift off on the airplane or at night when I can't fall asleep.

- Start with a mantra-based meditation.
- If you are feeling fatigued or when you reach the end of the mantra, simply roll off to one side and allow yourself the beauty of deep, restful sleep.

A meta-nap can accelerate healing and emotional wellness.

Candle Gazing

For very visual people, this type of meditation is quite easy, as they find it easier to let go of thoughts when they are concentrating on a physical thing rather than on a mantra. Especially for athletes—many of whom are visual by nature—this meditation can improve focus and concentration. I find that one in ten of my meditation students enjoy this meditation style the most. When you gaze at an object that captures your attention, you become totally absorbed and taken outside of yourself. Some people may find this meditation to be a bit of a challenge, as one has to keep one's eyes open and focused on a candle without blinking or watering up. With practice, most people find that they gradually become very comfortable with this type of open-eye meditation.

Candle gazing brings the mind to a place of stillness, distractions dissolve away, and the mind becomes focused on the flame. The candle gaze meditation is a performance-based way to improve your concentration and memory skills, and it can lead you into a deep state of clarity if practiced regularly.

- Light a candle and place it on a small table 3–4 feet in front of you.
- Sit in a comfortable posture with your spine upright and your arms and shoulders relaxed.
- Make sure that the flame is at the level of your eyes. Also, make sure that you are facing the candle directly without having to turn the neck even slightly. Try

to have a steady flame rhema (kindle) during the practice. Close the windows, make sure that there is no breeze of any kind to disturb the flame (turn off any fans or air conditioners).

- Take a few deep breaths to relax. Close your eyes and watch your breath as you inhale and exhale for 5–7 breaths. This will allow your breath to settle down and bring you into the present moment.

- Gaze at the flame intently and keep your gaze on it without getting distracted by outer disturbances and thoughts. Keep your vision focused and steady on the flame without blinking for 5–10 minutes. Try to avoid any kind of body movement during the entire practice.

Mental training plays a huge role in performance of any kind. The best mental discipline is the one you feel most comfortable in practicing and that generates the greatest positive results for you. Some athletes swear by visualization, while others favor various styles of meditation. Every person is different and possesses his or her own preferences and inclinations.

To unlock your true potential and go for the gold, the winning formula here is a combination of both visualization and meditation mental training.

ACKNOWLEDGMENTS

T hank you to the universe for giving me vision, to the fitness industry for giving me a home, and my yoga practice for constantly reminding me to practice more. Thank you to my teachers Renée Taylor and Dr. Lorene Hiris. Thank you to my mentor and adviser Jane Pemberton.

Thank you to Dr. Pam Peeke for giving me inspiration and a good role model. Thank you to Dave Coleman of the NFL. Thank you to my right-hand man, Scott Enright. Thank you to the YogaFit staff and trainers for doing what you do and keeping the vision. Thank you to the YogaFit network for believing in me, trusting YogaFit, and being so loyal. Thank you to my close friends who always have my back even when I don't. Thank you to my angels for showing up when I most need you. Thank you to my higher power for reminding me often that you are present.

INDEX

BETH SHAW, author, entrepreneur, and visionary, is the founder and president of YogaFit Training Systems, the largest yoga school in the world. Shaw is largely responsible for building the yoga market in the United States over the past twenty years. Established in 1994, YogaFit has trained more than 250,000 fitness instructors on six continents. The author of *YogaLean* and the bestselling *Beth Shaw's YogaFit*, Shaw has also created more than one hundred bestselling yoga and fitness DVDs and CDs. She is a sought-after speaker on topics of health, corporate wellness, women's business, entrepreneurial skills, and philanthropy. A lifelong spiritual seeker and student, Shaw is also an accomplished life coach, anger-management specialist, and meditation teacher. She holds a degree in business management from Long Island University and in numerous mind-body modalities. Of all her many accomplishments, Shaw is most proud of her philanthropic work and YogaFit's community-service initiatives. She sits on the board of many nonprofit organizations and is an outspoken animal advocate.

bethshaw.com
yogafit.com
@BethShawYoga

ABOUT THE TYPE

This book was set in Scala Sans, a typeface designed by Martin Majoor in 1994. It was originally designed for a music company in the Netherlands and then was published by the international type house FSI FontShop. Its distinctive shapes add to the articulation of the letterforms to make it a very readable typeface.